THE LAST OF THE BALD HEADS

Ferdia Mac Anna was born in Dublin in 1955. He has worked as a
television producer and director, journalist and magazine editor
and for some years toured Ireland as rock 'n' roll singer
Rocky De Valera first with the Gravediggers and then with
The Rhythm Kings.

Ferdia Mac Anna is married with three children and
lives in Dublin.

ALSO BY FERDIA MAC ANNA
Memoir
Bald Head (Raven, 1988)

Novels
The Last of the High Kings (Michael Joseph, 1991)
The Ship Inspector (Michael Joseph, 1995)
Cartoon City (Headline, 2000)

Plays
Big Mom (1995)
The Last of Johnnie Synge (1991)

Editor
The Penguin Book of Irish Comic Writing (Penguin, 1995)

The Last of the Bald Heads

Ferdia Mac Anna

Hodder Headline Ireland

Copyright © 2004 Ferdia Mac Anna

First published in 2004 by Hodder Headline Ireland

ISBN 0340 75239 4

The right of Ferdia Mac Anna to be identified as the
Author of the Work has been asserted by him in accordance
with the Copyright, Designs and Patents Act 1988.

A Hodder Headline Ireland paperback

1 3 5 7 9 10 8 6 4 2

A CIP catalogue record for this title is available from the British Library.

Typeset in Plantin Light by Hodder Headline Ireland
Printed and bound in Great Britain by Clays Ltd, St Ives plc

Hodder Headline Ireland
8 Castlecourt Centre
Castleknock
Dublin 15
Ireland

A division of Hodder Headline
338 Euston Road
London NW1 3BH

CONTENTS

To Kate, Sienna, Bessa and Finn
and to my parents, Tomás and Caroline.

Eldorado

Gaily bedight,
A gallant knight,
In sunshine and in shadow,
Had journeyed long,
Singing a song,
In search of Eldorado.

But he grew old—
This knight so bold—
And o'er his heart a shadow
Fell as he found
No spot of ground
That looked like Eldorado.

And, as his strength
Failed him at length,
He met a pilgrim shadow—
'Shadow,' said he,
'Where can it be—
This land of Eldorado?'

'Over the Mountains
Of the Moon,
Down the Valley of the Shadow,
Ride, boldly ride,'
The shade replied—
'If you seek for Eldorado!'

Edgar Allen Poe (1849)

1

Elvis Costello Saved My Brain

Dublin, 1985

The first thing I heard was a yelp.

I woke up in a white bed in a white room with the worst hangover ever. The sun blazed in through high windows turning everything in the room ghostly, stabbing fingers of light into my eyes.

I had a metallic taste in my mouth, as though I had been sucking an empty spoon. My teeth felt as though someone had removed them and stuck them back in upside down. I sat up. I felt stiff all over, and now I tasted blood in my mouth.

Opposite me there were two beds. In one, an old guy sat reading a paper. A teenage lad lay in the other bed, looking bored. Next to me was a white screen. Soft snores came from behind the screen. I tried to figure out what I was doing in a hospital bed, but nothing came. No memory at all.

Another high-pitched yelp. The yelps were coming from outside the room. Somebody must have brought their dog in, except that it didn't sound like a dog.

The yelps made me angry. Finding myself in hospital made me angry. Having no idea how I got there made me angry. Now I just wanted to get away. I wanted to go home. A new thought struck me – I don't know where my home is. I can't remember where I live. I can't even remember my name.

A milky nurse came over, looked at me and asked me if I was OK.

'Yes, I'm grand.'

'You sure?'

'I'm sure. Now go away, please.'

I didn't want her looking at me. I didn't want her asking me stupid questions. I wanted to ask her if she knew what happened to me, but I didn't want to look thick.

I was convinced that I had done something bad. Along with my anger, I felt guilty and confused. Nothing felt right. I didn't want to see anyone until I figured this out. I didn't want anyone to see me.

Milky Nurse said something else but I didn't get it. Either I didn't hear it properly or I just couldn't understand.

'Please go away.'

She shrugged and then walked off, consulting a chart.

Now I could get some peace.

A blonde woman walked in. She came over to look at me, face tight and concerned.

Immediately I felt mad at her. I didn't want anyone coming here to see me like this. I didn't want her looking at me either. I didn't want her asking me if I was OK. I recognised her. Her name was Maria.

'Are you—?'

'Yes, I'm OK,' I told her abruptly.

She said something but I ignored it.

'You don't have to be here,' I snapped at her.

'Do you know who I am?'

'Of course I do.'

'Who am I?'

'You're Maria.'

Maria looked shocked. 'That's what you were calling me last night. Who's Maria?'

I didn't need to be bothered with this now. Her name was Maria. She obviously had some kind of problem with her name.

Another yelp from the corridor.

I felt the urge to move. I had things to do, stuff to find out. I wanted to make sure somehow that nobody found out that I was in hospital. That seemed important to me.

Maria wouldn't let me alone. 'I've been outside all night. I'm really worried about you.'

'Well, you can go now. I'm fine. Don't tell anyone I'm in here.'

The word 'outside' scared me. Outside where? Outside this ward? Outside the hospital? Something bad had happened to me 'outside', but now suddenly I didn't want to know what it was. Everyone else seemed to know something I didn't, and that pissed me off. I wanted to ask Maria what had happened but I was afraid of what she might tell me.

'How are you feeling, Ferdia?'

'Ferdia?'

My own name came back to me, as though it was trailing a banner at the head of a parade of small memories. Ferdia. A sudden flood of recollections rushed through me because of that one word: I often got letters from people who thought I was a woman (for the attention of Ms Ferdia Mac Anna, the name sounded feminine); people had trouble pronouncing it (in London they called me Fred); I had grown up in Howth (in a little white bungalow near the top of the hill, just below the Summit Inn). I didn't think that I still lived there. I couldn't remember my parents or brothers or sisters, if I had any.

Then there was a sudden yelp from the corridor.

'Somebody give me my clothes and let me out of here. I want to go home.'

I knew that there was a reason that I couldn't go home to the little white bungalow in Howth. I could feel answers stirring deep within me as though trapped somewhere in my stomach. I could feel knowledge slowly working its way up my body until it evaporated somewhere just before it could pop into my mind and illuminate me. I couldn't understand it or rationalise anything. I was like a sheet of paper with some doodles and scribblings on it.

It felt strange not being able to remember, as though all of my memories had been wiped. Except for basic functions – like knowing what a fork was or recognising a window or realising that I was in a hospital bed – I was basically blank. I knew my name and I recognised Maria, but that was about it. The loss left me feeling empty and angry.

I wanted to blame someone for all of this.

The nurses pissed me off. The two blokes on the other beds pissed me off. The person snoring behind the screen pissed me off. The mystery yelper down the hall pissed me off. I wished that they would all go away and let me have a big think so I could work out what was going on. Except that I couldn't think. I couldn't figure anything out.

'Are you OK?' Maria asked.

'Yes.'

Maria's questions pissed me off.

I wanted Maria to go away and quit annoying me.

I closed my eyes and Maria disappeared along with the white room.

★

I woke up a few seconds later. Maria was gone.

In her place stood Milky Nurse, looking at me. 'Your wife will be back later, she's gone for something to eat. She was outside all night, you know.'

'My wife?'

'Yes, Kate.' Milky Nurse looked at me.

She asked the OK question.

'Of course I'm OK.'

'How many fingers am I holding up?'

'Two.'

'Now?'

'Four.'

'Good.'

The blonde woman was my wife? Kate. Not Maria. Who's Maria? Kate was American. We had met… I couldn't remember where I had met my wife. I couldn't remember getting married either.

My wife's name is Kate.

I was shocked to find myself married. I wanted to ask Milky Nurse if we had any kids but when I looked up she had vanished.

I shut my eyes. Tried to think. Nothing came. Better idea. Don't think. Shut down. Save the energy. Veg out on the hospital hum.

A yelp from the yelping man.

A nurse came in with a plate of dinner on a tray that she placed in front of me. I sat up and tried some. The food tasted like paste and I spat it into my napkin. I couldn't eat it. I rang a bell and when the nurse came I asked her to take it away. I asked her why the food was so crap. 'Is it always this inedible?'

'Well, everybody else likes it.'

She looked annoyed, but she took the tray away. Hospital food was crap.

Outside the windows, it was dark. I had a tight feeling in my head, as though I was wearing a crash helmet that was too small. I was awake but incredibly sleepy – except I couldn't sleep. I kept thinking but there wasn't much to think about because no more memories had returned. My mind was firing blanks.

I just lay there, listening to the hospital drone while counting the seconds between yelps.

The next morning Kate was back. She had the same tight look on her face. I asked her about the yelps. She told me the story of Yelping Man. It seemed the guy had been out jogging when he had suffered a sudden massive stroke. The last sound he heard was that of a dog yelping. Soon after he came to, he yelped. That's what he'd been doing ever since. Maybe he thought he was a dog. Kate said that he was in the next ward, sitting up in bed normal as anyone with his eyes open, giving a yelp out of him every thirty seconds.

Apparently, Yelping Man's ward was doing a big turnover in patients. Most lasted a day before asking to be moved.

'You're very lucky to be in here,' Kate said.

I didn't know what to say to that.

★

I refused to eat hospital meals. Everything tasted awful, even the toast.

I couldn't read or concentrate on anything for very long. I didn't notice days changing into night. I remembered mornings only because the white light was so bright through the windows that it poked my eyes awake.

In the morning, the old man in the bed opposite had gone. In his place was a man with a white beard. I recognised him – my dad knew him. More memories. My dad was a big man with a massive face. He could throw a deafening scowl if he was mad at you. Whenever Dad came back from America he brought me an album. Once I got The Doors, then it was The Flying Burrito Brothers. The best one and my favourite was *The Allman Brothers Live at the Fillmore East.* I remembered that I had a big record collection at home. I just couldn't think where my home was. I didn't want Dad to know that I was in hospital. I wanted to hear 'In Memory of Elizabeth Reed' by The Allman Brothers – it was my favourite piece of music. Listening to it always made me feel as if I was flying.

The man with the white beard had something to do with the Dublin Theatre Festival. I had met him several times. It triggered a new memory. Dad worked in the Abbey Theatre in Abbey Street, Dublin – a big, rectangular, ugly building. Outside on the side walls and in front of the main entrance posters of plays were displayed. I had spent a lot of time there as a child. I could feel Dad. Big man. Big presence. Schooldays when I would sometimes call into the Abbey for lunch money or a lift home. Dad sitting in the auditorium, directing actors on a stage. Dad's big, broad, dark back in the seat. The cigarette in his mouth, trailing wispy smoke up into the lights. Dad directing *The Plough and the Stars.* The standing ovation at the end. Dad directing *Borstal Boy.* The Tony Award on our mantelpiece at home. All those plates on the wall – those weird colourful plates.

I remembered being in the audience one night when all the lights suddenly dimmed and we heard a car approaching from the alleyway outside. Slowly, this ancient thirties jalopy drove onto the stage, its headlights gradually illuminating a group of actors who were dressed as Chicago gangsters. The remainder of the scene was played out in the headlights over the soft murmur of the car engine. Somebody got bumped off on stage. The lead gangster looked like Hitler. The title of the play jumped out at me: *The Resistible Rise of Arturo Ui* by Bertholt Brecht. Then the headlights switched off and my memories went into darkness. I chased the images for a while but got nothing more. It was as though titbits of memory were being filtered through, enough to tease me but not enough to lead me anywhere. I remembered that I had loved the play. That memory made me feel good for a while. I liked plays about Chicago gangsters. I liked old jalopies.

Mr White Beard got up, quietly put on his dressing gown and slippers and walked out of the ward. A few minutes later a nurse gently brought him back, helped him out of his coat and put him back to bed.

As soon as the nurse left, Mr White Beard got up again, put on his dressing gown and slippers and walked out purposefully, like he was going to a meeting. Moments later, the nurse led him back again.

This went on most of the night and the next morning. Mr White Beard didn't once make it past the end of the corridor.

★

Kate told me that I was supposed to remain in hospital for a few months until they had a chance to figure out what was wrong with me. They wanted to observe me and do more tests.

A few months?

No chance.

I wanted to go home.

I had a row with Milky Nurse over the taste of the tea, so she took it away. I refused to eat dinner and made a big fuss about it. I made a fuss about everything. I was obnoxious. Hospital food was crap and somebody should do something about it. Everyone else in the ward thought the food was fine.

In the end, it was decided that I could leave.

The nurses thought I was an arrogant shite and couldn't wait to get rid of me. They preferred the yelping man.

The next morning Kate came to collect me. I had everything packed.

Mr White Beard was standing by the side of his bed in his dressing gown holding a bag, just standing with a blank expression. He seemed to have lost interest in going anywhere.

Before we left the hospital, I wanted to see Yelping Man – I needed to put a face to the yelps.

We paused outside the next ward and looked in. Kate pointed out a normal-looking fellow in his late twenties or early thirties. There he sat in his bed. He looked perfectly normal, but he wasn't reading or looking at anyone. He just stared ahead as though contented.

We waited. He gave a sudden yelp. He made no big deal about it – it seemed like a normal thing for him to do.

We left the ward and walked down the corridor to meet my doctor. His office was small and murky with medical books stacked on the table, along with a bag of medical implements. The walls were covered with charts of the human brain and body. Neatly folded papers and forms lay piled on the desk. The doctor was an elderly skinny man with a quiet manner. He asked me several questions. He made notes. He held a small bottle with the cap off under my nostrils. 'Do you smell that?'

'Yes,' I replied.

Then I realised that I hadn't smelled anything. I was surprised. 'No,' I said quickly. 'I don't smell it.'

Alarmed, he removed the cap from another small bottle and put it to my nose. 'That one?'

'No.'

He made some more jottings. At one point he gave my knee a whack with a small hammer. He seemed relieved by my reaction.

He told us that he could not say for sure what had happened to me. The word 'aneurysm' was used. I didn't know what it meant. He explained, but I still didn't get it. The phrase 'spontaneous bleed in the brain' came up. I understood enough to know that I was very lucky to be alive and even luckier not to be a vegetable. Then I heard him tell Kate that there was some permanent brain damage. He said that there was a good chance of epilepsy.

Permanent brain damage?

Epilspsy?

I didn't believe him. I knew I was fine. I didn't want to hear any more. I wanted to get out of that murky room and get clear of the white rooms and the yelps and Milky Nurse and Mr White Beard and the quiet doctor as well. I shut out the doctor's voice. I didn't want to listen to the stuff he was telling Kate.

★

Kate drove us home to our small basement apartment on Crofton Road in Dún Laoghaire. As far as I was concerned, I had been in hospital for a few days and nights. In reality I had been in the public ward in St Vincent's for two weeks.

I recuperated at home for what I thought was a week, only it was really two months.

I had no dreams. Memories came back slowly, though some didn't come back at all. Nothing tasted good. It took me a while to realise that I had no sense of smell. I couldn't smell the dinner cooking or the toilet or perfume. I don't remember any visitors. Now and then something would trigger the memory of a particular smell, but it never lasted more than a second.

I was lucky. Things could have been a lot worse. If I had to lose one of my senses and I'd been given the choice, smell would probably have been the one I'd have picked.

Kate looked after me on her own while she continued working as a journalist for *The Irish Times*. I saw her walk past our bedroom door to the kitchen. I heard the kettle boiling and then tea being poured. Moments later, Kate walked past on the way to the front room and her typewriter. We were assigned no aftercare.

I knew I was also a journalist. I worked as arts editor for the *Evening Herald* but I had no memory of the job or of my colleagues. I still couldn't remember my parents or brothers or sisters. I couldn't recall my wedding to Kate. I didn't even know who Kate was. She was just there with me, my mysterious wife. I felt resentful of her. I wanted to blame someone for what had happened to me and Kate was the only one around – even though I knew that she was entirely blameless. My wife had saved my life and was now looking after me.

I was incapable of rational thought, and I immediately blocked out any emotion that frightened me or made me aware of my own fragility. I had no idea why I had called Kate Maria.

Sometimes memories just arrived unannounced.

I had grown up in Howth. I remembered long walks home from town whenever I missed the last bus – the number thirty-one. I had a friend called Nessan. We were two boys with weird names hanging around Howth together. My favourite soccer team was Crystal Palace. They used to have a centre-forward named Gerry Queen. One time he got sent off for fighting and the headline in the sports pages read 'Queen in Row at Palace'. I went to see the movie *Woodstock* when I was fifteen. Ten Years After were brilliant and I really wanted Alvin Lee's big red Gibson guitar with the peace sticker on it. Ritchie Havens kept strumming and strumming for ever and wouldn't finish his song. I really wanted him to get off the stage so that the next band could come on, but he just kept strumming. Even when he stood up to leave he kept playing. Irritated the shit out of me.

★

I couldn't read because I couldn't follow a train of thought. I watched television but had trouble concentrating or absorbing information. Often a programme would leave me behind after five minutes and I would be totally lost, unable to recall how it started or even what it was about.

I was grumpy all the time. I couldn't even enjoy music.

I was a nightmare.

Over the weeks, I pieced the day of my accident back together. I remembered being in the *Herald* offices and my work, typing up a film review. I remembered enough to make a story out of what happened.

It had started as a normal day. A columnist, Dominic Behan, wanted to meet me and Colm (the design editor and a good friend) for a lunchtime jar. We met him at noon in The Oval, next door to the Independent building. Dominic sat at the bar, under a portrait of his late, world-famous brother Brendan, though I don't know if he had noticed the portrait.

We drank pints. We talked. We laughed at Dominic's stories. He was living in Scotland. He said he felt accepted there and that he had never really felt accepted in Dublin. He was good company, but he got drunk quickly and turned bitter.

We went somewhere for lunch, or perhaps we walked around intending to go somewhere for lunch and then decided to go back to the pub instead.

I remember bumping into Nick O'Neill, the film-maker, outside Bruxelles. Nice guy. Big smile. We chatted to him a while before moving on. I remember bright sunshine in Grafton Street, like it was the start of summer.

We went to Larry Tobin's pub for another pint. Then, somehow, Dominic disappeared, Colm was gone and I was in a taxi.

Now it was night-time. I arrived at my friends John and Sally's apartment for dinner. I remember that Kate was annoyed with me for turning up a bit drunk. I denied being drunk. 'Just a few pints,' I said.

John and Sally had an old black pay telephone with an *A* button and a *B* button on the money box part. I showed them how to tap the phone so that you didn't have to put money in and then tapped out a call to my brother, Niall, and had a chat with him.

We sat at a table. I talked too much. A plate of spaghetti carbonara appeared in front of me. I kept talking away about something.

John put *West Side Story* on the stereo as I stood up to go to the toilet. A male voice sang about a girl named Maria.

That was the last thing I remember.

Apparently, I walked off towards the toilet only to collapse like an empty coat in the doorway. At first they thought I had passed out because of drink. They tried to wake me up but couldn't. I was completely gone. That was when Kate noticed that there was blood coming from my ear. She phoned an ambulance. She saved my life.

The ambulance arrived and they carried me out on a stretcher. I came to for a few moments on the stretcher. One of the ambulance men had recognised me from my time as a rock-and-roll singer. 'Don't worry Rocky, we won't tell anyone,' he said.

He thought I was drunk too. Everyone thought I was just drunk – everyone except Kate.

★

We went for walks. I couldn't remember much but I grew familiar with the small area between our apartment and the Dún Laoghaire Shopping Centre.

Sometimes we bumped into people we knew, though I never recognised them.

It was hard to tell if I was getting better. It took me ages to do the simplest task, like opening a can or boiling a kettle.

Then one day we saw a small man wearing glasses in a big overcoat walking in our direction. I thought I recognised him, but he passed without a sign or a nod that he knew me.

A few seconds later I knew who he was. 'That was Elvis Costello,' I said to Kate.

Kate was used to me rambling. I told her that I had seen him at the Stella in Rathmines around 1976. 'He was brilliant. He said that it was great to be playing in Dublin. That it was great to be playing in front of real people.'

I was very happy. I had recognised Elvis. He lived in our area. That was something I remembered from before. Everything was going to be fine now.

Elvis Costello had saved my brain.

2

Rock Hudson Could Have
Been My Daddy

My father met my mother on the set of a Rock Hudson film called *Captain Lightfoot* – a swashbuckling adventure about Michael Mann, an eighteenth-century Irish Robin Hood who gave the British a hard time in Ireland and America. The film was shot in 1954 in Ireland and Dad had a small supporting role playing the British army officer who arrested Lightfoot, played by Rock. In his big scene, Dad pointed a pistol at Rock and delivered the line, 'Take this man to the captain.'

A framed colour still of this moment hung on the wall in the front room of our house in Howth when I was growing up. There was Dad looking stern in a red coat and a tall hat while alongside him stood Rock Hudson, appearing unperturbed at being surrounded by bristling redcoats. Rock Hudson was disguised as a monk.

Mother played an Irish rebel. Her big scene was shot at Bective Abbey, where she stood in the midst of a gathering of irate Irish insurrectionists. At one point she raised her fist and yelled, 'Up the rebels!' She doesn't appear in the film again. She always maintained that there was a lot more to her role and a good deal more dialogue, but her scenes had been dropped because of 'politics'.

Mother's rebel hung on the wall next to Dad and Rock. Dressed in an Irish rebel costume of long skirt and a shawl, she looked wan and enigmatic as she posed in a doorway.

Dad fell in love with my mother the instant he saw her on the set and told his friend that he was going to marry her. Dad's friend told him he had no chance, but Dad's friend was wrong. Dad asked Mom for a date and she said yes.

At this point, Dad began to notice that Rock was taking an undue interest in my mother whenever she was on set.

Rock called Mom Caroline. Mom called Rock, Rock.

When the movie wrapped, there was a big ceilí for the cast and crew. Rock Hudson asked my mum to dance, so she taught him the 'Walls of Limerick'. They appeared to be having great fun, which made my father angry. He wasn't having this Hollywood star muscling in on his girl.

At one stage my father went eye-to-eye with Rock. Words were exchanged. For a brief moment, it looked as though Dad was about to burst Rock Hudson, but common sense prevailed and someone intervened. There was no punch-up.

Rock Hudson returned to Hollywood where he enjoyed a successful movie career, unhindered by the fact that *Captain Lightfoot* was only a minor hit. (In the seventies it inspired Michael Cimino's *Thunderbolt and Lightfoot*.)

A year later, the British redcoat and the Irish rebel got married.

It was a pivotal time for my parents, and maybe for young

Rock too. For a brief moment back in 1954, had Rock considered abandoning his closet life as a gay man for a shot at heterosexual happiness with my mother? Could I have been the son of Rock?

Not according to my mother's version.

She said Rock was never around and, anyway, she didn't fancy him. He was too namby-pamby for her tastes. She also said there was no confrontation at the ceilí. She might have had one dance with Rock, but there was no threat of Dad bursting anyone.

The real problem on set was jealousy. According to Mother, others grew envious of her auburn hair and striking good looks. This explained the mysterious disappearance from the finished film of all but one of her scenes, and was also the reason her dialogue in that scene was cut back to just one line.

When I was a kid, the Lightfoot story made perfect sense. I liked the idea that my parents had met in such an incredibly romantic way. It was how true love should be.

I used to tell people that my parents had fallen in love on a movie set. I thought it made me special. Basically my parents were Hollywood folk, or they could have been if they hadn't given up the cinema for love. They had starred in a movie with Rock. I may have added that Rock always sent Christmas cards and never forgot a birthday. Sometimes, for a dash of added colour, I bragged that I might have been Ferdia Hudson – even though Ferdia Hudson doesn't sound like a normal name, it's a lot easier to pronounce than Ferdia Mac Anna. Everyone always pretended to be dead impressed.

The more I talked it up, the more true it became.

I stuck with Rock Hudson throughout my childhood and teenage years and into my twenties, thirties and early forties.

Then, in March 2001, Dad published his autobiography and swept the legacy of Rock Hudson out of my life. Written in

Irish, *Fallaing Aonghusa* is my Dad's account of his life in the theatre, and it contains the official version of how my parents met.

In 1954, Dad worked in Radio Éireann and one day he was standing in the lobby waiting for the lift. He had a script under his arm – a play in Irish that he'd written for the radio. Then the lift doors opened and a tall, slender woman walked out. Dark and striking, the woman carried herself with a majestic air.

Dad was gobsmacked. He fell in love the instant he set eyes on this *speirbhean* – because she was literally a woman from the skies.

He forgot about the lift.

He watched the auburn-haired woman walking away and thought about her for the rest of the day and all night.

The following morning, he was sitting in a café on O'Connell Street with a friend when the woman from the skies walked past. His friend commented on her beauty and Dad said that he had it in his mind to marry her. 'You'll never do it,' his friend said. 'You're too busy to be chasing women, even a beauty like that girl.'

Dad bet him five pounds that he would marry the girl and the friend said he looked forward to pocketing Dad's fiver.

Dad then had to find out the identity of the woman – who she was, where she was from, where she worked. He thought that she might be an actress with the radio company. He set out to track her down. For a while he had no luck and began to think that he had seen a vision rather than a real woman. But eventually he got a tip-off from a friend that she worked in the General Post Office. Her name was Caroline Sheerin and she worked as a secretary of some sort and was interested in acting.

Now all Dad needed was a strategy. He considered just walking up and introducing himself, but decided against it for fear that it might be too presumptuous. He thought about phoning her, but dismissed that as too distant. In the end he decided to write to her. He wrote her a note introducing himself and inviting her to audition for a pageant he was producing.

After waiting a couple of days – which seemed like an age to him – he heard back from her. She would be happy to meet him and she would be interested in auditioning for the pageant. They arranged to meet in a cafe in Westmoreland Street.

They met and Dad bought the *speirbhean* a cup of tea.

Before half an hour had passed, he told her that he wanted to marry her without delay.

There was a moment between them.

She told him that she was going outside to buy a packet of cigarettes and have a bit of a think. She went outside and smoked and thought things over while Dad sat in the café and fidgeted. After a short time, she came back in and said that she had decided that it was a good idea to get married. Dad's reaction to the news is not recorded.

That night, to celebrate their engagement, he took her to see a play. Before long, Mom was cast in a pantomime called *Blaithin and the High King*, a reworking of *Cinderella*. Later, they worked on *Captain Lightfoot*, where Dad may or may not have come close to bursting Rock Hudson.

Since Dad's autobiography was published, my parents have denied the story about meeting on the set of *Captain Lightfoot*. However, the photograph of Rock and Dad still hangs in my parents' house, alongside that of the Irish rebel girl. Nowadays the movie story sounds like showbiz fantasy, whereas the *speirbhean* story has the ring of truth.

I know which one I prefer.

In our house there was a story about everything and it was often difficult to tell which stories were made up and which were real. In the end, I gave up trying and went with whatever story sounded the best. Truth and fantasy amounted to more or less the same thing – it just depended on how good the story was and how well it was told.

My parents' stories made me feel uncertain about the world, though. Anything you believed could be changed by a story. I liked stories that were written down in books or told as movies or comic books. These stories were solid. I found it easy to believe in John Wayne and James Bond and Ray Bradbury and even *Just William* because these stories always stayed the same. Nevertheless, I accepted my parents' stories as true at the time they were told. As a kid, it never occurred to me to doubt them.

I was born on 17 August 1955, about a year after *Captain Lightfoot* was made. Nobody remembers what time it was, but Dad reckons that it was early afternoon. It was a protracted birth – Mother said that I took my time before popping out – and a year later I was baptised Tomás Ferdia Mac Anna.

For reasons that are not really clear, nobody ever called me Tomás. However, there is a story about it, one that I carried with me for a long time and on a sunny day when the world seems a bright and happy place, I still believe it…

On the day when Mother suddenly had to go into hospital, Dad was in RTÉ directing a radio play called *Ferdia and Cúchulain* – or it may have been *Cúchulain and Ferdia*. The play told the tragic story of the mythical Irish hero Cúchulain, who because of 'politics' was manipulated into fighting his best friend, Ferdia, by the devious Queen Maeve. After a three-day battle, honours were even, so Cúchulain resorted to dirty tricks – he stabbed Ferdia through the heart with a magical Gae Bolga (a short spear that could not be diverted from its target) and then held his dying friend in his arms. Afterwards, overcome with grief, Cúchulain tied himself to a rock by the sea and died of heartbreak and remorse.

The play was broadcast live with an actor called McKenna playing Cúchulain – nobody remembers who played Ferdia. I was born halfway through Act One.

During the break, McKenna was called aside and given the important telephone message that his wife had just given birth to a baby boy. Mother and child were healthy and doing fine. McKenna looked surprised. 'That's incredible,' he stammered. 'She's only six weeks pregnant.'

In Act Two, Cúchulain's performance was lacklustre. He appeared to be preoccupied. During the climactic battle it looked as though Ferdia was going to win but, after vigorous and audible prompting from the wings, Cúchulain remembered his Gae Bolga and Ferdia was slain.

Cúchulain emerged victorious but traumatised. People said that the mythical hero's final distraught speech as he tied himself to a rock and prepared to die was quite moving, though it was apparently largely improvised and contained very few of the original lines. Afterwards, they found out that the message was intended for my dad – I don't know if anyone bothered to tell McKenna.

Dad rushed to the Hatch Street Private Hospital where he found his wife and newborn son. He named me Ferdia after the noble warrior who gets bumped off by his best friend.

The name Ferdia means man of the Fir Bolg and anyone who says different is spoofing. There are various other translations – including 'man of God', 'iron warrior' and, my favourite, 'man of smoke'. Dad said he had often wondered why Ferdia was so little used as a boys' name, but when he tried to christen me, an old fuddy-duddy priest objected to a child being given a 'pagan' name. To appease the priest, Dad stuck Tomás before Ferdia and joked that I'd be the first St Ferdia – it didn't quite turn out like that.

Nobody ever called me Tomás – not even Dad – so Ferdia stuck.

My dad's first gift to me was to name me after a mythical loser whose name sounds, well... feminine. Not quite a 'Boy Named Sue', but close enough. He condemned me to a life-time of spelling my name down the phone to people.

Nevertheless, I'm glad he didn't call me Cúchulain – I wouldn't have wanted that much weight on my shoulders.

3

The Independent Republic of Mom

I was three when I nearly bumped off my mother.

I was playing on the carpet of our house in Killiney. There was no furniture in the room. Instead, there was a cardboard box filled with shiny white three-prong plugs. I thought the plugs looked and felt wonderful. My little sister and I played with the plugs for a long time, but she was little and not much use at games. She was more hair than human – her ringlets got in her eyes and she toppled over a lot. I had given up trying to play with my sister when Mother walked into the room so I decided to play with her instead. I threw her a plug, thinking that she'd catch it and come over to join in the game, but the plug smacked her in the face and hit the floor with a *thunk* just before Mother collapsed.

That was when Dad walked in. He gave me a terrifying, deafening glare and looked like he wanted to throw me out the window. 'You could have killed her!' he roared.

The plug-thrower was picked up, put somewhere and left to wail. The box of plugs was removed and stuck in a high cupboard.

For years I believed that I had almost assassinated Mother. Now I can't tell for sure if the plug throwing ever really happened, though I can still vividly recall the arc of the plug as it tumbled though the air towards Mother. I can still hear the *thunk*.

This memory is a story, a distillation of my parents' memory and mine, continuing the family tradition of storytelling – giving me another memory to be uncertain about. Perhaps it is merely a product of their invention. Maybe I imagined the whole thing after some dream. Today it makes no difference whether the plug story is true or not because the tale is stuck in my head for ever. I still resist any opportunity to change a plug. If I am forced into it, I make the change as quickly as possible, plug in the lamp or record player or television and then scarper. I move away from the scene of the plug in case it might bring disaster.

In our first house in Killiney, the rooms were small and seemed to have no furniture. Every room had pale walls.

When I was a baby, Mother tried to get me to say my first word. She said the same thing to me over and over again, hoping that I would mimic the sound. 'Massachusetts.'

My attempts to say the word made her peel into laughter. 'Massachusetts,' she'd say.

'Mama-Chu-chuf,' I'd say, and Mother would crack up.

She'd call Dad and say the word and again I'd repeat my version and Dad would crack up too. Big booming laugh. This went on for ages, maybe for weeks, until I got the word right.

I liked making Mother happy. I liked making people laugh. I liked being the centre of the universe.

When I was older, Mother often told me the 'Massachusetts' story. She explained that she wanted my first spoken word to be difficult so that every word that came after would seem easy.

Like most people, I have few memories – reliable or otherwise – of being a baby. I can remember sitting up inside a big black pram facing down Killiney Hill, looking out at the vast blue sea. I recall being terrified of a pair of stone lions that adorned a gateway on Avondale Road. I always put my hands over my eyes as we went past and could not be reassured that the lions were simply stone decorations. The lions were real to me; they were just lying in wait.

I felt an intense, scary weightlessness as the pram trundled downhill, bouncing me towards a Martello Tower. I thought that a ghost lived in the tower, which was actually a sweet shop. Mother bought me a fig roll that I bit into and immediately spat out. This wasn't a sweet, it tasted more like medicine. I couldn't eat it. Some man took it from me and made a big show out of munching it, making faces that were intended to show me how good it was and what I was missing. I wasn't impressed. If adults wanted to eat fig bars, then let them.

★

My best friend in Killiney was Peter Green, who lived nearby. We played together most days. I was four when our family left the house in Killiney to move into an apartment in the city, though Mother promised that she'd bring me back every weekend to play with Peter – but she never did and I never saw him again. Perhaps she meant to bring me back to Killiney to play with my friend, but forgot. Maybe it was just a promise made to smooth over the moment of departure, but I couldn't understand why Peter had suddenly disappeared from my world. I couldn't understand why my parents couldn't fix the problem. I felt a terrible sense of loss, made worse because it was unexplained.

Many years later I moved back to the southside, to a house less than a mile from our first home in Killiney. Once, when she was visiting, Mother claimed to have met Peter's mother. Peter was a merchant navigator at sea. Apparently he still remembered me and for a long time after I left expected me to return to play with him at weekends.

Our new home was a flat in a side road off Pearse Street, the darkest street in Dublin (At least I remember it as Pearse Street, my dad says it was nearer Stephen's Green). All the buildings on the street were murky and dingy-looking except for the theatre where Dad worked. The theatre was called the Queens, but was really the temporary home of the Abbey Theatre, which had burnt down years before.

Sometimes I was brought into the theatre to sit in one of the boxes and watch Dad direct plays. Once he put me in the box overlooking the stage where the carpenters were fixing scenery. 'Stay quiet now. I'll be next door. I have to chastise someone,' he said. A short time after he left me, I heard movement next door. I listened as intently as I could as he admonished an actress for consistently showing up late and not knowing her lines. The woman tried to charm him, but his voice remained calm and controlled. He told her she was on final notice – if she messed up again, she was out.

Dad bought a cine camera as well as a Bell & Howell 8mm film projector from Hall's Photographic Shop in Talbot Street. The shop was filled with 8mm movies; many of them specially edited silent versions of contemporary films. I asked Dad to buy me *The Blob*, starring Steven McQueen. He said he'd think about it. (A year or so later, Dad gave me *The Blob* which had been cut down to around ten minutes. It was one of the silliest, least scary horror films ever made, but I watched it incessantly. Dad often watched it with me. We agreed that it was a truly dreadful movie, but we kept watching it because it was ours. I loved the flickering noises of the projector and I adored putting a sheet over the curtain rail to turn our front room into a mini movie theatre.)

Later he began filming inserts in the flat for a spoof on James Bond novels for an Abbey pantomime. In one sequence, an actor dressed as Bond came up the fire escape and in through our window. He chased a villain around our flat and back out onto the fire escape, where there was a mock punch-up that looked nothing like the real thing. There were no sound effects, just grunts and someone whispering instructions. 'Now fall over there, go on. No, no – on the flat part.'

Later they blew up a car in the alleyway outside our flat – or rather, they threw something into a Morris Minor and smoke hissed out. It was very unconvincing, even to a four-and-a-half-year-old.

I asked if I could use the camera to make my own film, but Dad shook his head. 'Wait until you're older,' he said.

On the first night of the pantomime, the film was projected onto a big backdrop to loud music theme. It looked quite exciting. I was just getting into it when it ended abruptly, seconds after Bond jumped through the window of our apartment. The screen went to black. Suddenly, the lights came up on stage to reveal the Bond guy crouched below the projection screen, as though he had just landed. What followed was colourless in comparison. The Bond guy was far more exciting and interesting on screen than on the stage. Once the film was over, the rest was just dull old theatre.

The next day, I went out into the street to play with some local kids. We found a box of matches and decided to blow up the Morris Minor for real. There couldn't be much to it, we reckoned. Just light a match and toss it in the gap between the slightly open window and the roof.

I was the oldest and tallest so it fell to me to light matches and toss them in. The matches landed on the seat and went out.

Then I remembered something I had seen in a film. Some guy had thrown a lit match into the petrol tank of a car and caused a spectacular explosion. That was what was needed here – a spectacular explosion. Then maybe Dad would give me a job in the next film he shot. I could be in charge of blowing things up. I just needed to show him that I was good at it.

So I lit a match and slowly removed the petrol cap. The other kids gathered round. I held the match close to the silver hole where the petrol went in. I could smell the petrol fumes. The others shouted encouragement, 'Go on, Fergi, go on. Do it.'

I threw the match at the hole but it hit the side of the nozzle and fell onto the tarmac, where it went out. I tried again. Same result. Then we only had one match left.

I went close to the hole and lit a match. This time I would stand right beside it and shove the lit match in. I looked in and smelled the acrid petrol fumes. There was definitely petrol in the tank.

I struck the last match and it flared. I pushed it at the hole, but I did it too fast and the match went out just before it fell in. We stood around for a moment and wondered where we might get more matches.

Then Mother called and I ran in for dinner.

★

After living in the apartment for a year, we moved to Howth. Our new house was a whitewashed bungalow near the summit that stood at the end of a long driveway. From our front porch I could see acres of bumpy green fields sloping down to the blue sea and Ireland's Eye beyond. The air was so sharp it hurt to take a deep breath. It was like living on top of the world.

The house itself was small, but I got a bedroom of my own. So did my sister. There was a front garden and smaller rockery garden just below the front porch. In the garden sat an old rusted roller that I wanted to flatten things with. I was disappointed to find that it was so decrepit that it wouldn't budge.

There was also a big back garden and lots of fields of rolling grass and heather with a hill of broken rocks beyond that looked ideal for war games. Everywhere was green and wild. The place made me want to put on sneakers and run.

There was an important difference between the bungalow in Howth and the house in Killiney (I can't remember much about the flat in Pearse Street except that it had a big window overlooking a fire escape). The bungalow had furniture. There were chairs and tables in the kitchen and dining room as well as a sofa in the front room.

On the first day, the local kids came around to check us out. 'Where are you from?' one asked.

'We come from the High Kings of Ireland,' I replied, repeating what Mother had told me to say.

The kids were not impressed. A girl said that she was going to ask around about us. She reckoned we were from Cabra.

I was five years old. My sister was three and a half. I didn't like the new place and during the next fifteen or sixteen years I never warmed to either the house or the beautiful location. Perhaps I missed my friend Peter, or maybe I just didn't want to live on top of the world, where it was cold and windy and where everything seemed to be either uphill or downhill with no flat surfaces.

Not long after we moved to Howth, I met Nessan in the doorway of the summit shops. 'Give me two pence or I'll burst you,' he said. I wouldn't give him two pence, so he burst me and I ran home crying. A few days later, Nessan and I gave up fighting each other and became friends instead. He was skinny with fair hair and sharp features and was the first boy I had met who was as tall as me. Nessan's people had lived in Howth for over a hundred years. (Anyone whose Howth roots didn't go back at least half a century was regarded as a 'runner in'.)

We formed a gang and hung around the shops. We played football, robbed orchards and cycled our bicycles at dizzy speeds along dangerous cliff walks and rattly back paths or *bóthareens*.

When we were eleven or twelve, our biggest kick was to freewheel down the Hill of Howth to the town without using brakes. Sometimes we managed the feat with arms folded. We steered with our feet on the handlebars. We were lucky. Nobody got hurt.

★

One winter the family got mumps. I was nine or ten, my sister was eight, my brother Niall was four and our baby brother Naoise was around a year old (my sister Darina was born about a year and half later, thus completing the family). 'You all look like Richard Dimbleby,' Dad said. We all thought it was hilarious going around with puffed-out faces.

But Naoise got really sick. I remember the doctor arriving late one night and I heard Naoise coughing in my parents' bedroom. Later Dad brought him to hospital. I saw the red tail lights of the Austin Cambridge disappearing down the driveway.

Naoise had meningitis and was in a coma for six months. When he woke up he had permanent brain damage. Mother took us into the study to tell us about our brother. She was strange; there was something missing from her voice, which sounded flat and tired. Naoise was lucky to be alive, she told us, but he would be four or five years old for the rest of his life. His body would grow up, but his brain couldn't because of the brain damage. 'Unless there's a miracle,' Mother said. 'You can never rule out a miracle.'

Naoise came home from hospital. At first I didn't notice anything different. He was still just a little kid. But once he began to walk around, he had to be watched all the time. He liked to wander off. He spent a lot of time at the Summit Inn, chatting in his jovial and limited way to people drinking pints outside. Sometimes we found him in the shop, loading up with chocolate bars.

Throughout my childhood and teenage years, Naoise escaped all the time. Whenever I found him at the Summit or in someone's garden he smiled and gave me a big hello.

Sometimes he liked to sit at the end of the driveway and toss rocks out into the traffic. Luckily he never caused an accident and people were usually very gracious about it whenever he bounced a rock off their bonnet. They could see that he was an innocent.

On other occasions he disappeared completely. We'd often get a phone call to pick him up from someone's house or garden. Sometimes we searched for him in vain, only for him to simply reappear a few hours later without us ever finding out what he had been up to.

Though we were ostensibly Catholics, I rarely heard any mention of religion in our house and we never went to mass. The only times I recall going to the big Catholic church in Howth town was for funerals and the time I made my Holy Communion. If the neighbours were concerned about us, they never let on. Howth was either a liberal and tolerant place or Howth people were really good at keeping their feelings to themselves.

Mother decided to bring Naoise to Lourdes. She told us that people with all kinds of disabilities had been brought to Lourdes by their loved ones and returned home miraculously cured. 'Lourdes can miraculously cure Naoise,' she said.

'But we never go to mass,' I said.

'Of course we do,' Mother said. 'We are always there in spirit. God knows that.'

'But Lourdes is a place for believers,' I continued, recycling some knowledge I had picked up in school.

'I'm a believer,' Mother said.

Mother and Naoise went off to Lourdes the next morning. When they came back Naoise was still the same, miraculously uncured.

By the time I started college, Naoise had gone to live in the first of a succession of special facilities for autistic people. He still came home at weekends and he always enjoyed going for walks, but he rarely wandered off anymore and he had long since given up tossing rocks into the traffic.

★

In the summertime, Dad went away to lecture in US colleges or direct plays in Berlin or Newfoundland or on Broadway in New York City. He went off to a working life that we could not imagine. He sent back letters from the US with dollars in them. It was exciting to get crispy dollars in the post, but the letters only came now and again and the money was quickly spent. Dad was gone all summer and to me as a small boy it seemed like for ever.

Theatre was Dad's other family. In many ways it was a more important unit for him. Mother said that she was only his mistress and that theatre was his wife.

We went on family holidays once, and only once, for a week to Butlin's in County Meath. I don't recall any birthday parties in our house. We got birthday presents and a cake at teatime and that was it. The best birthday present I ever got was a sleek blue-framed Raleigh bicycle. Dad had picked it out for me. 'It's a tall bicycle for a tall boy,' he told me.

One Christmas, Dad dropped all the presents while trying to leave them on my bed. 'Shag it,' he said, and I woke up. I asked him why he was picking up all the presents in the doorway. Why hadn't Santy left them on the end of my bed as he always did? 'Santy got tired,' Dad said. 'He left them in the hall.'

That was how I put two and two together about Santy. It's

also the only Christmas I remember.

When Dad was away we fought for possession of his big black leather easy chair in the study. Most times, because I was the oldest and the biggest, I won. But I could never sit comfortably. The chair was too wide and the leather felt strange. It squelched beneath me whenever I shifted my weight.

But the real frustration was that I could not get the footrest to work. I couldn't get it to go *yang*. A big leather easy chair without a working footrest was a disappointment. I yanked at it and even jumped up and down on the chair, but got no joy.

One day, I broke the footrest. I couldn't budge it. I was terrified. The big face would glare down at me. The big voice would boom in anger.

For the rest of that summer, I sat anywhere in the study but Dad's chair. My brother and sister didn't bother with the chair once they saw that I wasn't interested anymore. A pity, since I was keen to find a way to blame the damage on one of them.

At the end of that summer, Dad came home from the US. I dreaded to think what was going to happen when he discovered that someone had banjaxed his footrest. He had a rage on him sometimes. He could shout at you and you felt like you'd been lashed by a hurricane.

I had decided to plead ignorance. I knew he wouldn't believe me and, even if he did, one of the others would squeal.

Upon his return, Dad walked into the study and stretched. Then he sat down on the black leather easy chair, which groaned. He got comfortable, and then he leaned back.

I held my breath.

There was a brief *yang* as the footrest popped up under his feet, as perfect as before – as though he'd never been away.

When Dad wasn't around Mom coped with things at home, but she often yearned for Dad. She waited for the weekly phone call from the US, which always lifted her for days afterwards. She had to deal with five kids with no car (Mother didn't drive anyway), no help and a husband who spent a huge amount of time in the theatre or else working abroad. She always told us how tough it was. She told us that she needed us to behave ourselves as 'little adults' until Dad came home. She didn't want to have to write to Dad or phone him to tell him that we were causing her grief. We'd get no more letters with dollars in them if she did that and we would be in big trouble when Dad came home. She told us that her nerves were bad after the trauma of Naoise. The doctor had advised her to drink Guinness to keep her strength up. She was a lot more distant after Naoise's illness, as though some of the lights behind her eyes had been dimmed or switched off. I got into a lot of arguments with her, perhaps because I felt neglected. Whenever I grew frustrated after rowing with Mother, I picked on my younger siblings, especially my little brother Niall, who I deeply resented because Mother had moved him into my room without my permission or even a consultation.

Sometimes, when Mother was feeling down, we kids got together to make her laugh by telling jokes or acting out stories or imitating TV programmes or movies we'd seen. Niall was the best mimic; he could make anyone crack up, no matter how tense the situation. I always felt better when Mother was smiling or laughing. As long as we could keep her amused, we would have a happy house, I thought. We seemed to have happy times and sad times with no in-betweens. I couldn't imagine what it must be like to have days or weeks or months where things happened quietly or smoothly or without incident. I couldn't imagine what it must be like not to be blamed for bad behaviour or disgracing the family or other atrocities. I learned to shut down whenever Mother blamed me for stuff. Even when I was guilty, I taught myself not to feel.

Mother smoked a lot of cigarettes. I got used to being sent to the Summit for two bottles of stout and twenty Carroll's. Other days she sent my sister. We usually brought Naoise with us for the walk – at least then we knew where he was.

One day I held Naoise's hand as we walked down Thormanby Road to Howth town. It was a beautiful sunny day. The sky was blue. We were going for a long walk to the shop by the church in the town to buy sweets. Then we would take the bus back up the hill. I was twelve. Naoise was three or four.

A tall man with grey hair fell into step alongside us and he began to chat to me. I didn't say much – I wasn't sure if he knew me or not. Perhaps he knew my parents. He appeared friendly.

He invited us to go for a walk down the tram tracks with him. He said it was very nice down there. I said we couldn't. 'We're going home,' I lied.

'Excuse me,' the man smiled. I noticed that he spoke with a lisp and that he had an iron tooth in his mouth. 'Does the young boy wear bway-ces?' He didn't wait for an answer; he leaned over me and pulled up Naoise's shirt. I pulled Naoise away. 'It's easier without bway-ces,' the man smiled.

I said nothing. I kept walking down the hill holding Naoise's hand. I didn't know what was happening. I didn't have words for it. What did he mean? What was easier without the braces? I felt scared, but I kept walking.

'I could do it if I wanted to, you know,' the man said. 'It would be easy.'

I looked ahead for anyone I knew, but there was nobody about. It seemed like a long way down to Howth town. I wanted to find an adult that I knew. I wanted to get away from this strange man.

The man may have said something else, but I don't remember. I remember the sound of our footsteps and the warmth of Naoise's hand in mine. Naoise hadn't noticed anything amiss – his shirt still hung loose behind him where the man had pulled it out from his trousers. I kept trying to plan what I would do if he touched Naoise again or if he put his hands on me. I considered walking into a house and knocking on the door, pretending it was where we lived. But if there was nobody home and the man hung around, I might end up trapped in someone's doorway. It felt safer to be on the footpath in daylight.

Somehow, we reached the town without anything else happening. I turned left at the church and the man kept walking straight ahead without breaking stride or saying anything. I went to the sweet shop and bought sweets. It was all I could think of to do. We walked to the phone box outside Howth Library, keeping an eye out for the man, and then I rang home. 'I think we've been attacked,' I told Mom.

I don't recall if Dad came to collect me or if we took the little red bus home. I sat in the black easy chair in the study and told Mom the story and she phoned the police.

A few hours later two policemen arrived and took a statement from me. I told them all I could remember. They were very interested to hear that the man had an iron tooth and a lisp and they kept asking me about his tooth.

I never heard any more about it.

★

At home, I rarely felt relaxed around my mother. There was always something going on between us. I felt that I could do nothing right – that I was excellent at doing things wrong.

She told me that she wanted me to be well behaved.

She needed me to do something for her.

She was always disappointed in me for messing or giving cheek.

She wanted me to be nicer to my sister and to quit beating up on my little brother.

She needed me to stop disgracing the family when we went outside the house.

But when people were around, things were different. Outside the shops, she sang my praises to people she met. I heard her on the phone telling someone what a gifted and polite child I was. At the Abbey on a first night, she held a crowd hostage with details of my brilliant drawing. She told everyone how talented I was – neighbours, painters and decorators who came to our home, friends of Dad's, actors and writers and stagehands and lighting guys, the Russian ambassador, the Papal Nuncio, the milkman.

But I didn't recognise the person she was describing. Quite often I had acts attributed to me that I had never performed or could not recollect. I had helped so-and-so across the street. I had won a prize in school for History (the only prize I ever won for anything was a small square of Connemara marble with a seagull stuck on it for coming first in 'Find the Sod of Turf', a game at Irish college one summer when I was thirteen). I was brilliant at reciting poetry. I had taken great care of my sister. On Sunday mornings, I cooked breakfast and served it to her in bed.

It was as though some alternative fantasy son with a brilliant career as a goody-goody was being managed by Mom. It made me apprehensive. I always felt tense around her, as though I was expecting to get dropped into an embarrassing situation, like being told to recite a poem or show people my drawings and read from the little red cashbooks in which I wrote stories.

Mother loved talking about this fantasy son. The only problem was the actual presence of me, her real-life son. She must have noticed my discomfort because she usually sent me off to do something so that she could continue praising her fantasy boy.

I picked up on some of the words she used to describe me. 'Noble' and 'honourable' were huge ones. 'Loyal' was another biggie. They all meant the same thing: always do as Mother says and don't give her any cheek.

I noticed that people praised her whenever she told them about her kids. Dad got praised and received awards for directing plays and coaxing magnificent performances from actors. Mother picked up imaginary Oscars for detailing the achievements of her children.

I often felt as though I wasn't a real person, merely a prop for Mother's 'performance', something to help her get attention and praise. I never identified with any of the labels she put on me, though I tried hard to be 'noble', which seemed to involve standing around quietly while my mother spoke to other adults. I learned to switch off whenever Mother made me the centre of attention for things that I had not done and other stuff that I couldn't relate to. But it pained me that I couldn't live up to the publicity. Fantasy son definitely led a more colourful and rewarding life. Fantasy son had a better relationship with his mother. Fantasy son had talent and grace and composure under pressure and kindness in abundance. Fantasy son was perfect. When she got nowhere with me, Mother gave up and switched her attentions to my sister and brother. I don't know how they felt about becoming fantasy kids, but they seemed to cope with it better than I did. I went around surly and quiet, afraid to open my mouth in public.

★

Mother charmed people when she was in the mood. She liked painters, writers and actors. She loved to encourage the young creative types in the neighbourhood. I grew accustomed to coming home from school and finding a young artist of some kind drinking tea in the kitchen while Mother gave him advice on his career. One landscape painter brought her new work every couple of days. She told him he should have his own exhibition. I know who to ring, she said and went out of the room to use the phone in the hallway.

'She's right. I deserve my own exhibition,' he told me grave-
ly. 'Your mother is a great woman.' I figured that she was
knocking around with this eejit because she was disappointed
in the real me.

I didn't bother trying to compete. I gave up drawing and
painting because I didn't want to find myself being compared
to any of Mother's friends. Instead I retreated into books. I
read and re-read Ray Bradbury stories. I found more comfort
and reality in fantasy tales than in my own life.

One Bradbury story, 'The Homecoming', became a particular favourite. The story's hero, Timothy, is a fourteen-year-
old boy growing up in a large extended family composed of
vampires, werewolves, clairvoyants, winged uncles, telepathic
little sisters and other strange and spooky beings. Timothy's
problem was that he was normal – a situation that greatly disappointed his mother and father, who kept expecting him to
'change' to become one of them. Timothy couldn't drink blood
and was afraid of the dark. He would give anything to be
accepted as a full family member rather than being regarded as
an interloper. I identified with Timothy's frustrations and was
particularly captivated by the boy's relationship with his
favourite relative, Uncle Einar, a huge man with great wings
who travelled by night. At one stage, Einar gave Timothy a
taste of what it was like to be to be a normal member of the
family when he took him flying.

I would not have minded if it had turned out that Dad was
a winged beast from the old country who sprouted wings and
travelled abroad several times a year to feast on the blood of
mortals. I wouldn't have worried if Mother had turned out to be
some kind of clairvoyant telepath. My young life might have
made more sense then, to me at any rate. I found great solace in
weird and wonderful stories. Books were a great place to hide.
Whenever I read them I could let my feelings fly. I wished that I
could have had an Uncle Einar, but in his absence I contented

myself with tall tales such as *The Illustrated Man* and *The Martian Chronicles*.

Mother seemed to be loved by everyone. People stopped me on the way home from school to tell me that my mother was a 'great woman'. I accepted that Mother was a 'great woman' to other people. I could see that she had greatness in her by the natural way she took charge of situations and also by her ability to get people to do things for her. I thought that there must have been something wrong with me because I didn't get on that well with her. I figured that I mustn't be a very nice boy. My good, normal personality traits must have got lost somewhere or else they had never arrived.

★

Mother liked to make a dramatic entrance. She could make getting out of the passenger seat of a car look like she was dismounting from a royal carriage. She had a natural glow about her. It was something in her blood. She never let us forget that she had been an actress. She loved to 'appear' in a doorway or at the top of a flight of stairs and immediately catch everyone's eye, striding forward with her thin, pale hand extended. 'I'm Caroline,' she'd say. She stuck close to her husband, but she could operate alone if necessary. She seemed to have boundless confidence and to radiate a compelling integrity and sense of joy. 'I am someone special', her presence said. People gravitated to her and she always held them spellbound. On first nights at the Abbey, Caroline and Tomás were like the President and First Lady of Theatre, and I was their firstborn son.

It was impossible not to watch her when she was in the same room. She was striking and slender and elegant. She dressed in dark colours that offset her auburn hair – and her hair was auburn, never red and definitely not brown.

As well as charming people, she could also manipulate them

when she wanted to. Once I had a toothache and had to stay home from school, so she decided to take me to the dentist. She phoned to make an appointment, but the dentist was booked up that afternoon. 'This is Caroline Mac Anna of the Abbey Theatre,' she announced. 'I want to make an emergency appointment for my oldest son. I have been informed that you are an excellent dentist. Is this information correct?'

The dentist fitted us in right away. I could hear her talking and laughing with him in the next room as I sat in the dentist's chair with my mouth open, waiting for my gums to be excavated. Immediately before inserting a needle filled with anaesthetic into my gum, the dentist told me that my mother was a 'great woman'. I wasn't surprised.

The local taxi man in Howth was named McConkey. He was a round man with an impassive face. Whenever Mother wanted to get anywhere she called him and he always came, even if she had no money. She ran a slate, which she paid off every so often. He never complained.

★

As I grew older, I often felt a need to challenge mother's assumptions, and this meant rows and disagreements. Mother developed a habit of saying 'imagine that' if she was losing an argument or felt boxed into a corner. After a time, this was shortened to 'imagine' and could end up a contemptuous snort of ''magine' if things grew heated.

Once I argued with her over some trivial matter. She got tired of arguing and walked away. 'You have no feelings,' she told me.

Her dismissal made me very angry. 'Yes I do,' I shouted. 'I do have feelings. Lots of feelings.'

'The Bible says that the son who raises a hand to his mother will watch that hand wither.' That stopped me.

'But I haven't raised my hand to you.'

'You raised your voice and that's the same thing.'

Some days Mother was fine. Other days she acted as though she was fed up and couldn't be bothered. I found her changes of mood bewildering. I felt off-balance and awkward around her. When Mother was in a bad mood, my defence was to become monosyllabic and gruff.

One of my friends had asked his mother about sex and had been told some balderdash about pollinating flowers. I decided that I would ask Mother, partly to find out the answer, but also just to see what might happen.

One evening I stood outside the open bathroom door while she was looking at herself in the mirror, putting on her new earrings. 'Mother, what's sex?'

She froze. Her fingers paused with an earring halfway to her right ear. 'What?'

I repeated the question.

She shrugged. 'It's a religious thing. It's sacred.'

'But what is it?'

She slowly adjusted her earring. 'I told you,' she said and brushed past me. She carried on into the study, where she closed the door.

'But you haven't answered my question,' I shouted.

'Imagine,' she called back from behind the door. 'Look it up in the dictionary.'

I looked up sex in the various dictionaries, including the *Encyclopaedia Britannica*. The explanations were always dry and unenlightening. In the end, I found out some basic facts by talking to friends in the schoolyard.

The disagreements also embraced politics and nationalism. Mother thought all the British soldiers who were in the North of Ireland should be shot or driven into the sea. The Irish army had chickened out when they had the chance. Now it was up to the IRA. I told her that the IRA soldiers were not real soldiers, they were cowards who shot people in the back.

'Hah,' she said. 'And what would you know about it?'

I said I thought that killing people in cold blood was wrong.

'What have the Brits been doing to the Irish for eight hundred years, eh? Answer me that?'

She listed British war crimes against Ireland. Bumping off the leaders after the 1916 Rising was evil, but shooting Connolly while he was in a wheelchair was worst of all and proved that the British had no morals. She thanked God that I was attending an Irish-language school.

I pointed out that most people in Ireland spoke English, including our family. She gave a hollow laugh. She told me that I must think that I was very clever. She told me that Ireland unfree would never be at peace. I replied that we were free down south, in the independent Republic of Ireland.

'Yes,' she said. 'I might have expected you to say that. And I am free in the independent Republic of Me. Freedom is just a word. It means nothing until you are walking your own sacred land and speaking your own tongue.'

I gave up arguing with her.

★

Another aspect of Mother's personality was her tendency to launch into sudden, dramatic stories just when you were at your most tranquil. One night she came into the study, where I was watching television. She told me to turn off the television. She had an important announcement. I switched the TV off.

It was about Dad's plane from St John's in Newfoundland. One of the engines had gone. They were trying to make it to an airport on one engine.

I stood up. I didn't know what to do. Did this mean that Dad's plane was going to crash? 'God willing they will make it,' she said. She told me that I could go back to watching TV. I sat there for a while. I turned on the TV because I couldn't think of anything better to do. I kept thinking about Dad's plane flying on one engine. How had Mother found out about it? Maybe the captain had phoned relatives from the cockpit, just in case.

About an hour later, she came in again to say that the plane had landed safely. She asked me to say a prayer in thanks. Dad was a bit shaken, but he was fine and he would be home tomorrow.

I couldn't sleep that night. I was confused about air travel and plane engines in particular. I had watched movies where pilots had made it back to base after being shot up on an air raid. This was the first time I had heard of a plane engine just cutting out. What if *all* the engines cut out simultaneously on the next plane Dad took? It could happen.

Dad came home the next morning. When all the welcoming had died down, I asked him if his plane had had to crash land in Newfoundland. He looked puzzled. He told me that there had been no problem on his flight.

Later, I asked Mother about the plane engine cutting out. 'Just be glad he's back home safe and sound,' she said.

It had never occurred to me that Mother might have been making the whole thing up, perhaps for attention because she felt lost and lonely. I figured that there must have been some truth in the story, but I don't know why she did it or if anything dramatic had actually happened on Dad's flight from New-foundland.

One night, a few months after the 'Newfoundland' incident, I lay in bed shivering. The night was freezing and I didn't have enough blankets. I was too tired to get up, but too cold to drop off to sleep. The bedroom door opened and Mother appeared in the light from the hallway. I pretended to be asleep, but I kept one eye partly open. She took down my big black school coat from its peg on the back of the door and walked across to my bed. Carefully, she spread the coat on top of my blankets. Immediately I felt the extra weight pressing down on me and I felt warmer and more secure. Then Mother went over to check on my little brother in the bed across from mine. After that she padded softly to the door and went out, closing the door behind her, leaving the bedroom in darkness. It was one of the few times in my childhood that I felt truly cherished.

★

At home, Mother never discussed her childhood or mentioned anything of her family history. It wasn't until I was an adult and had to fill in insurance forms that required extensive family details that I realised that I didn't even know her maiden name.

It was as though her history began the day she met Dad.

However, she had no problem relating stories about our ancient family mythology. She said we were descended from the ancient kings of Ireland. 'Why do you think we called you Ferdia?' she asked me. 'If anyone asks where you come from, tell them you come from the High Kings of Tara.'

Once she told me that I had Spanish blood. One of her ancestors had become 'involved' with a survivor from the Spanish Armada. Most of the men on the Armada ships that shipwrecked off Irish shores either drowned or struggled ashore only to be slaughtered by the British or sometimes by the locals. One bedraggled Spanish soldier had washed ashore and somehow made it inland as far as Leitrim. There he had been discovered by my ancestors, hiding in one of their barns. Apparently, our Armada survivor was visited that night by a curious female relative who wished to see what a real Spaniard looked like. The Spaniard and the Armada groupie got on so well that they were discovered naked in each other's arms the next morning, whereupon the story turned either murky or tragic, depending on your viewpoint.

The Spaniard was either bumped off by outraged ancestors or betrayed to the Brits. Either way, he was never seen again.

Nine months later the female ancestor delivered a Spanish Armada baby. Mother maintained that the baby must have been a girl because there were no Spanish surnames in our family. (Until the seventies, and the unexpected arrival of Rocky De Valera. But that's another story.)

Anyway, I believed that we had Spanish Armada blood in our family well into my thirties. Then, one day, Mother casually admitted that it was all only a tall tale. I was astonished that she could casually demolish a truth that I had held sacred for ages. I had felt comfort in feeling that I was somehow connected to the Latin world. Now I was plain old Irish again.

Despite my age, I grieved. Without Spanish blood in my veins, I felt oddly undiluted.

4

An Underpants of Acid Drops

The Christian Brother appeared suddenly from behind the wooden partition. He carried a small boy sideways like a battering ram. The boy's legs stuck straight out behind him, pale and stiff like a turkey that had just been lifted out of a freezer. At the top of the classroom the Brother adjusted his grip, then abruptly and repeatedly slammed the boy's head into the blackboard. White chalk dust rose into the air like gun smoke as the blackboard trembled with each slam.

My class watched the incident through the half-opened wooden partition doors that separated our classroom from the large Georgian room next door. We had been left unattended to await the arrival of our new teacher. The Christian Brother from the class in the next room was supposed to be watching over us. His idea of minding us was to crash some kid head first into a blackboard.

This was my first morning in Coláiste Mhuire, my new school.

Dad had dropped me off that morning at the school entrance. It had taken us ages to drive into town from Howth. He said I was going to one of the best schools in the country and I felt brand new in my new school uniform.

After the fourth or fifth slam, the Christian Brother said something in Irish that I couldn't understand before dumping the boy roughly on the floor. Shakily, the boy made his way back to his seat.

Fifty nine-year-old boys sat still as statues, trying not to give the Brother any reason to come into our classroom to pick out one of us for blackboard duty. For a long time we waited in silence, not even daring to whisper to each other. We stared into space or examined our schoolbooks. When the partition door between the classrooms closed softly, we began to breathe properly again.

We heard voices on the other side of the partition and the sound of another door closing, followed by footsteps in the hallway outside our classroom. The footsteps drew closer to our room. Our classroom door opened and a tall dark Christian Brother whose eyes were hidden behind thick black glasses stepped into the room. He said nothing. He just looked us over for a moment. His face was calm as the water in Howth Harbour on a windless day. We were all relieved that we weren't going to have to deal with the Brother next door. But this tall man – whose nickname we soon found out was Bruiser, a variation on his surname in Irish, which was unpronounceable – still looked a bit dangerous. He seemed offended by having to be in the same room as a bunch of kids. Standing there that morning glaring through thick glasses, he scared the shit out of me.

Coláiste Mhuire was an Irish-language school for boys and at that time was the only such school in Dublin. The Brothers appeared certain that within a few years everyone in Ireland would be speaking Irish as a first language. Kids came from all over the city – from Cabra, Whitehall, Portmarnock, Malahide, Blackrock, even as far away as Dunboyne in County Meath, such was its excellent reputation – I was the only one from Howth.

Every school morning from the age of nine, I got up at seven, dressed and had breakfast and gathered my stuff. I waited at the bus stop across the road for the little red bus to take me down the hill to the Howth train station, where I caught the train into the city. Getting off at Connolly Station, I walked up Talbot Street and O'Connell Street to Parnell Square. I seldom met anyone I knew during these journeys. I left home before the local kids rose for school and nobody in Coláiste lived out my way. The other northside kids took different buses or got a lift into school with their parents.

I was very lucky, Mother told me that morning at breakfast. Coláiste Mhuire produced only the best future leaders of the country – lawyers, politicians, soldiers and revolutionaries. You couldn't make anything of yourself in Ireland without having fluent Irish. Coláiste Mhuire would make a man of me. She made it sound very exciting.

On the first morning, it didn't take long for the excitement to disappear and be replaced by a deep feeling of dread and unease, one that lasted throughout my time in the school.

That first morning, I wished that I had never left St Fintan's in Sutton, where I had spent Second Class.

★

I had always loved reading and books, but I had never been a great student.

I started in Howth National School when I was five. It was a flat grey building, located up a leafy side street from the town. Most mornings my father drove me to school, dropping me at the entrance. By the time I was seven I was making my own way to school and back home, either by walking down the hill or catching the little red bus. The first, and in many ways most important, lesson I learned in Howth National was that Howth was a town, not a village. That lesson was explained to me by a boy named Jim as he and his pals held me face down in a pool of mud in the field behind the school. I never forgot it.

By the time I was in First Class it had become obvious that I was weak at maths. I was moved to a double desk to sit beside a boy named Colm, who was the best in the class. The teacher must have thought that some of Colm's brilliance would rub off on me; instead it was the other way around. My lack of numerical ability frustrated Colm. He had been used to being named best student on a weekly basis. He and his previous desk-mates had scooped the various weekly prizes – usually Dairy Milk bars or bags of Tayto. Now I was holding him back. He couldn't understand why I was so mediocre at maths.

One day Colm decided that he would come home with me to see where I lived. He lived in the town and I lived near the top of the hill. He wanted to see if it was true that people from the town were smarter than those from the hill. After school, I walked to the bus stop outside Howth Library while Colm dashed off home to get changed.

As I waited for the little red bus, I prayed that Colm wouldn't show up. I didn't want to bring him home with me. Colm may have sat beside me in school, but he wasn't my friend and you only brought friends back to your house. Also, I had not invited him to visit me at home. He had invited himself. Even at my young age, I took exception to that kind of presumption.

The little red bus came and there was no sign of Colm. I got on, paid my fare and took my seat. I deliberately avoided looking out the window in case I saw him. As the bus began to pull away I felt happy and relieved, but immediately there was a sudden lurch and then the bus stopped. The doors opened and Colm climbed on board. He saw me and waved, paid his fare and made his way down to where I was seated. He seemed to be sucking something. He sat beside me and asked me if I wanted a sweet. Reaching under his belt he rummaged in his underpants before producing a bag of acid drops. I told him I didn't like acid drops.

At home, after an awkward bus journey, Colm introduced himself to my mother, who was delighted at his cheek and confidence. He met my sister and my baby brother, explored our back garden, checked out the back fields and then he came back inside our house and politely requested to see my bedroom. Reluctantly, I brought him down the hall and showed him my room. I managed to hide my teddy bear, Jojo. Colm was very taken by the James Bond pictures that I had carefully removed from an annual and stuck to the wall with Sellotape. However, he insisted that he had better ones at home, claiming to have a wall-sized poster of *Doctor No*.

Colm stayed until just before teatime before announcing that he had to go. Before he left to catch the little red bus, he told me that he didn't see any reason why I couldn't be as good in school as he was.

After First Class I was moved to St Fintan's in Sutton, which had a playground that overlooked a beach. I sat behind Leo, who had a crew cut and a magnificent booming, cultured voice. Leo was always picked to read passages from books or recite poems. When my class was entered in an annual Feis Scoil, we were all forced to learn off a dreadful poem called 'I Bounce My Ball'. Leo, though, was given a complex alliterative poem about pots of jam and other delights. The idea was that Leo would dazzle everyone with his booming voice and win while the rest of us mere mortals would achieve a kind of benign uniformity that would show the school in a good light.

On the day of the Feis, I clammed up. My shyness destroyed my performance. I stood on the stage and whispered the lines I could remember, hoping that nobody in the vast darkened hall would hear me. I was glad that my parents weren't there. We spent most of the morning seated at the side of the stage, watching as hundreds of kids from various schools recited, 'I bounce my ball/I bounce my ball/I bounce my ball most every day.' Finally, Leo came on and recited his pots-of-jam poem, drawing huge and prolonged applause. Leo won the competition. Afterwards, on the way home in a special school bus, Leo told me that he wasn't interested in poetry at all. He much preferred space rockets. 'One day, I'm going to be an astronaut,' he said.

My best friend in St Fintan's was a smart, jolly boy named Seymour. Perhaps we became pals because we both had an unusual first name. We hung around together and grew very close even though, for some reason, we were in different classes. One morning we came back after a break and the teacher told us that there had been a terrible tragedy – Seymour had dropped dead during gym class. We were to say a prayer for him, which we did.

I didn't fully grasp what was going on. I was supposed to go to Seymour's house after school to play, or perhaps he had been coming to mine. I had some of his toy soldiers in my house and I wondered whether it was right to give them back or keep them. Apparently Seymour was now in the gym room, laid out on a table. I wanted to go and see him, but the teacher told me that it wasn't possible.

At home I told my mother that Seymour was dead, but she was busy tidying up or getting ready to go out to the theatre. For whatever reason, she didn't discuss it with me.

So I sat down and watched television. I was confused and heartbroken, but I couldn't cry for my friend. I wasn't sure what death really meant. I couldn't grasp that I would never see him again.

When we left our old house in Killiney, I lost my first friend, Peter Green, but Peter was still in Ireland, as far as I knew. It was just that I never saw him or played with him anymore. Where was Seymour? I knew that young people weren't supposed to die. Old people grew older and eventually passed away peacefully in their sleep and young men got killed in wars or in shootouts with secret agents or policemen. Heroes always got shot in the arm and recovered quickly. Sudden death was usually for baddies. That was about all I knew about death. Both my grandfathers had died before I was born, so their passing meant nothing to me. At that stage, I hadn't even seen a dead animal up close.

I don't recall Seymour's funeral. Perhaps I didn't go or wasn't let go. Maybe my parents were trying to protect me or perhaps in those days it wasn't considered healthy for children to attend the funeral of a friend. Seymour was never mentioned again, either in school or at home. It was as though he had never really existed except as an imaginary friend. Seymour and Peter Green, my two best friends, had been removed from my world without explanation. I began to feel that this was what happened to those you grew close to. One day your friends simply vanished. I wondered when it was going to happen to my friend Nessan, even though he seemed too strong and tough to ever disappear.

Many years later, in my early thirties, while I was working as a film reviewer for a national newspaper, I attended a press screening for a new Irish film. A crucial scene was set in a graveyard on the Hill of Howth. The camera slowly panned across a series of gravestones to find a group of characters standing at an open grave. For a few seconds, the camera showed a close-up of Seymour's gravestone, displaying his full name with dates of birth and death. I went numb – my traditional reaction whenever I was in shock or felt a danger of my emotions rising. I had not thought about Seymour for many years and now here was his gravestone in gigantic celluloid close-up.

I felt bad for never having visited his grave to say goodbye. I felt guilty for never having cried.

★

Coláiste Mhuire was based in a large Georgian building situated on the corner of Parnell Square, approximately twelve miles from Howth.

Bruiser terrified us during his year as teacher of Third Class. Though he never hit me, I saw him use the leather strap on boys at least once a week. Once he produced a bamboo cane to administer a dozen cracks across the hands to some poor lad. I wasn't particularly good at lessons, but I wasn't the worst in the class either. For some reason, perhaps because I was quiet or maybe because my father directed the school pageants, Bruiser left me alone. An awkward and bespectacled boy named Wigglesworth was given a hard time because of his surname. It was as though Wigglesworth had committed a crime just by showing up in an Irish-language school with a handle that was obviously foreign – or worse, English. After a while Bruiser gave up attempting to put Irish on Wigglesworth's name during morning role call. Each morning, Bruiser called out the names for us to answer '*anseo*' ('present'). Bruiser silently ticked the names on his list. Whenever Wigglesworth answered, Bruiser snorted.

I felt lost in Coláiste Mhuire during primary school. There were too many boys, at least fifty in my class, and the teaching was abrupt and dismissive of anyone who couldn't keep up. I learned to keep my head down and not draw attention to myself. I was rarely called upon to read or answer questions or recite tables. All teaching was conducted through Irish, a language that I found difficult and frequently baffling. Even English lessons were frequently interspersed with bouts of Gaelic. Because I couldn't grasp the Irish, I fell behind in geography, history, maths and other subjects, especially languages.

I felt as though I had been thrown into an alien, unfriendly and exclusive environment. I pretended I knew what was going on, but at least half the time I really hadn't a clue. I was too shy and scared to ask for help or extra tutoring. I didn't want to risk a belt of the leather.

Luckily the boys all spoke English to each other between lessons and at break. The threat of expulsion hung over anyone who was caught speaking English and we heard stories of older boys who had been unceremoniously dismissed for speaking the 'alien tongue'. Soccer was banned, as were rugby, rock music and long hair. Gaelic games such as hurling and Gaelic football were mandatory. Handball was considered Gaelic and there were handball alleys in the schoolyard.

We learned 'Irish dancing' as part of our school activities. A tall theatrical woman with a worried face taught us jigs and reels, but she had grave difficulty controlling fifty high-energy boys who used dancing as an excuse to try to knock each other over. One afternoon when as usual the lessons had dissolved into anarchy, she broke into English to inform us solemnly in her resonant theatrically trained voice that unless we mastered 'The Walls of Limerick', none of us 'would ever find a decent woman to marry'.

Outside school, everyone I knew spoke English – even my parents, who had insisted on my attending Coláiste Mhuire. I don't remember my parents ever asking me how school went or what kind of a day I'd had. Maybe they did, but I have no memory of it. Perhaps I made my feelings known to them only to be ignored. More likely, like most kids in those days, I just accepted what was happening and got on with things.

I survived primary school in Coláiste Mhuire by never volunteering for anything and staying out of trouble. I didn't get into any serious fights and I mixed easily with the other boys. I remained wary of making close friends. I didn't want to meet another Seymour or Peter Green.

In Fifth Class we were taught by a huge, roly-poly, pipe-smoking lay teacher named Burke. Burke always wore a tweed jacket and was rarely seen without an unlit Sherlock Holmes-type pipe dangling from his mouth.

Burke had a very short fuse, but he often left us alone for long periods. He liked to set us a task and then sit at the top of the class to chew his pipe and read his paper. He did not like to be disturbed. Burke ignored me. I don't recall having anything much to do with him during the course of the year. One day somebody plucked up the courage to steal Burke's leather when he was out of the room. A bunch of us went to the edge of O'Connell Bridge after school and ceremoniously tossed it into the Liffey. Within a week Burke had got himself a shiny new leather strap. I wondered if there was a factory somewhere that manufactured these things, or perhaps the Brothers made the weapons themselves as a warped labour of love.

Most of us watched the punishments meted out by some of the teachers with a kind of morbid fascination. Violence was what happened to you if you screwed up your homework or were caught messing. There was nothing we could do about it. That was the way things were.

★

Despite's our fear of punishment, a bunch of us started an Authors' Club. There were three principal members – myself, my friend Pádraig and Pádraig's best friend, Killian. We sat at the back where, because there were so many kids in the class, it was usually possible to hold meetings of our club without being noticed by Burke.

Members of the Authors' Club wrote short stories in red cashbooks. We wrote the stories after homework or at weekends and then passed them around to each other for comment. We discussed our latest works in class whenever we got the chance. We wrote direct, uncomplicated all-action and deeply heroic tales that were inspired by our favourite films or TV programmes: *The Man From UNCLE*, *Combat*, *Have Gun Will Travel*, *Gunsmoke*, *The Twilight Zone*, *The Invaders* and James Bond films. Heroes tended to be straightforward, upright and in the employ of some shadowy agency that was dedicated to the preservation of the free world, or at least what we knew of it. The stories often climaxed with a gunfight or helicopter chase or a bout of fisticuffs that lasted for several pages and occasionally comprised over half the story's length. There were very few, if any, girls in these stories.

I always included an author's message on the first page of my red cashbooks. I welcomed readers to my new story or collection of stories and often warned them of the reading experience that lay ahead for them, particularly if there was excessive violence. 'I am sorry but I had to put it in because of reality,' I wrote in one opening address. Sometimes I provided updates on the condition of a hero from previous books. 'I am happy to say that Agent Matthew has nearly recovered from the harpoon wound.' I usually inserted an intermission in the middle pages in which I drew portraits of the heroes or characters from movies and I also used the page to plug my upcoming works – '"Five Mad Mexican Gunslingers" will be ready next month.'

I frequently recounted lame schoolboy jokes, possibly in the certain knowledge that the heroic tales contained in the cashbooks were short on laughs. The last page was always reserved for a personal thank you to readers and often included a list of my previous titles with advice to new readers to check them out by contacting 'the author'. I liked the idea of being an author. I reckoned that writing about heroes would be an excellent job for when I left school.

In the beginning, every story from the Authors' Club was an object of wonder and curiosity to the members. We each greatly admired one another's work. There was praise and harmony and our numbers grew. We set high standards – boys who wrote *Famous Five*-type adventure stories were not encouraged to join. We didn't want those types in our club.

The first controversy came after I wrote a story called 'Satan's Saint', about a gunslinger that happened to be possessed by the devil. My gunslinger alternated between bouts of extreme heroism and deranged murders. The Authors' Club was deeply divided about this story, with lively whispered discussions at the back of the class. The general feeling was that I had committed a crime against storytelling by writing such a weird and unbelievable tale. Whoever heard of a gunslinger that had been possessed by Satan? I was asked if there was a history of devil worship in my family.

I was proud of my story. I liked writing about a bad guy who didn't know what he was going to do next. The story had been easy to write. In fact, it had just seemed to write itself. This gunslinger didn't have to be truly accountable for his bad actions. In a strange way, I felt that I wasn't truly responsible for my gunslinger. The gunslinger had just somehow arrived in my head, fully formed. I didn't think there was anything weird in his being possessed. Maybe a lot of bad guys were possessed by dark forces. As far as I was concerned, that would explain a lot of things.

The negative critical reaction didn't put me off or get me down. Instead it inspired me to write a sequel. In 'Satan's Saint Part Two', the possessed gunslinger, Luke O'Dell, is tracked down and finally captured by Sheriff Paul Hindman – a real cowboy character hijacked from the *Pictorial History of the Wild West* that I had been given for Christmas. In jail, the gunslinger protests his innocence, having no memory of the murders. At the end of the story, the gunslinger is shot by Sheriff Hindman, but the possessed bad guy dies an innocent with no memory of his evil deeds.

'Satan's Saint Part Two' was a complete break with established Authors' Club practice. It was even more controversial than the first story. It was unrealistic, Pádraig said. Amongst other things, he complained about the relatively few gunfights and the fact that the bad guy represented both good and evil. This time the criticism hurt me. I thought that a writer should be able to write whatever they wanted. I figured that having a gunslinger possessed by the devil was every bit as realistic as any James Bond adventure.

When Pádraig passed his new story around, I made sure to hammer it. Unfairly. There was nothing really wrong with Pádraig's new tale, I was just paying him back for having a go at mine. Criticism of one another's works now became the dominant force in the Authors' Club. The reviews were often savage.

The Authors' Club changed from a mutual-appreciation society to a group of competitive eleven-year-old ego-maniacs. Pádraig and I and several others used the morning meetings to tear each other's work to ribbons.

Killian, a small thoughtful lad who loved to go bird watching, always tried to make peace. The irony was that Killian's excellent and quite lyrical stories were often overlooked or underappreciated in the jousting between the other founder members of the club.

One day Pádraig accused me of plagiarism. I had written a story called 'The Sea of Jelly', an overblown *Man from UNCLE*-type romp about a fiendish plot to hold the world to ransom by a villain who possessed a chemical that could turn the oceans into jelly (an idea lifted from some spy novel I'd read). At one stage the boss briefed the hero and announced that the chief suspect was a mysterious villain named Baron Nog. Pádraig had objected to this sequence on the basis that it was virtually identical to a story of his that had been circulated several weeks previously. Pádraig's spy had also been briefed by his boss about a mysterious baron called Nib or Nub or something similar. Pádraig and I argued. Which came first? Baron Nib or Baron Nog? Neither of us would back down. Killian intervened, but even his quiet diplomacy was useless. Outsiders were consulted for their opinions. The club fell apart in acrimony. Rival clubs were set up, but after a while everything petered out. I swore to never associate with other authors again, it was too much hassle.

However I kept writing, though I don't know if the other members of the Authors' Club did. After primary school we were separated into different classes. I never spoke with either Pádraig or Killian again except for a brief 'Hi' if we happened to pass in the corridor or bump into one another in the school-yard. I didn't like to admit it, but I missed the Authors' Club. I missed the attention and the sharing and I missed being a member of an exclusive club. I even missed the mad arguments.

★

By the end of Sixth Class I had amassed over sixty red note-books with stories in them. One night I came home to find Mother reading my red cashbooks. She told me that I was a genius. She boasted that she would get them published in the US. She had contacts in McGraw-Hill publishers. They would probably pay me a couple of hundred thousand dollars for my stories. She was putting the stories into the post as soon as pos-sible. In the meantime, she wanted to take legal advice to make sure that I got what was due.

Soon afterwards I came home from school to find a small cheerful man sitting in the front room with my parents. His name was David and he was a lawyer. Mother had showed him my stories and, though he had not had time to read them prop-erly, he could tell that they were very impressive. He wanted to take me out to Dún Laoghaire Pier to discuss what our next step should be.

Somehow, the following Saturday afternoon I ended up in

Dún Laoghaire with David the Lawyer. I don't recall how I got there, but I must have taken the bus or train from Howth and travelled across to the other side of Dublin Bay to meet this odd friend of my mother's who had taken a shine to my stories and was going to help my 'career'. We walked up and down Dún Laoghaire Pier in the freezing cold for what seemed like hours. He talked about what he was going to do to sell my stories to a US publisher. None of what he said made any sense to me. It grew dark quite suddenly and I began to feel uneasy. Why had my patents allowed me to meet up with this weirdo? Why did I have to travel all the way to Dún Laoghaire? Why couldn't we have met on Howth Pier?

I began to grow afraid. I told David the Lawyer that I wanted to go home and he was disappointed. He offered to put me up in a hotel, but I insisted on leaving right away. I walked to the bus stop and he followed behind. He travelled with me into the city. I remember that we sat on the top deck and that he kept rabbiting on about my work, though it had become clear to me that he hadn't read any of my stuff. In town, he walked me to the thirty-one bus stop and then waved me goodbye.

I never saw him again.

5

My Brilliant Acting Career

Halfway through rehearsals for the school play, the director (who happened to be my father) grew frustrated at the inability of a couple of shepherds and Mary, Mother of Jesus, to follow simple instructions and exit stage right instead of stage left. After yet another cock-up, Dad sighed softly and said 'Fuck' into the microphone.

Instantly, Mary, Mother of Jesus, and two dozen ten-year-old-boy shepherds froze.

The Christian Brothers who were overseeing the school production suddenly turned away, seemingly preoccupied with their own thoughts. Everyone stood still as statues, lest the slightest creak should provoke another bad word. The only sound in the hall was a gentle crackling from the PA system's massive speakers.

Dad sat in the middle of the empty auditorium with his lips pursed, as though about to whistle a tune.

This was Dublin in 1965.

Nobody ever swore in front of ten-year-old boys, let alone a bunch of Christian Brothers and certainly not during rehearsals for a school play about the Resurrection of Christ. We listened to my father breathing into the microphone.

I was a Roman soldier. My directions had been to stand at the side of the stage, holding a long wooden spear in front of me while keeping a menacing look on my face. I had developed a menacing look backstage in the bathroom mirror. Narrowing my eyes to slits, I had then curled my lip into what I thought was a forbidding sneer. I had seen a villain do something similar on *The Man from UNCLE*. I was proud of my menacing look but now I had a pain in my face from holding the expression for too long.

I wasn't among those who had messed up their exits. I was mortified and yet in a way proud that my dad could bring everything to a standstill. I had never realised that a word could have such impact. I decided to ignore the pain and hold on to my menacing look. I didn't want to give Dad any reason to single me out. Finally, Dad scratched his head. 'OK, let's do that again.'

This time there was no problem. The shepherds and Mary, Mother of Jesus, exited stage right as instructed and the rest of the rehearsal ran smoothly.

Outside in the yard at break time, I was mobbed. 'Did you hear what Mac Anna's dad said in the new hall?'

'His dad said "fuck".'

'In front of the Brothers.'

'It was massive.'

My popularity soared. Boys came up to me to ask if my father spoke like that all the time in front of Christian Brothers. 'Did I know any other bad words?' 'My father worked in the Abbey Theatre. They must say "fuck" all the time in that place.' 'Was life at home pretty fierce?'

Keen to capitalise on my new-found popularity, I told everyone who wanted to hear that my father said 'fuck' at home quite a lot. He even said it on Sundays. I told them he threw plates and forks. Once he had thrown out a goldfish bowl with the goldfish in it. It had taken us ages to find the goldfish in the backyard and we'd had to put the goldfish in a soup bowl.

The reception was so gratifying that when I ran out of remembered stories, I made stuff up. I told them that the previous Saturday Dad had lost his temper and torn a front wheel off his car with his bare hands. My audience of ten-year-olds swallowed the lot.

Even the ones who hadn't been in the hall took my word for it that my father was a wild man.

One boy suggested that I write down all the bad words that my father had ever said. We could make a list. That way, when someone annoyed us we could consult the list to pick a bad word to say or to call someone. We made a circle in the yard and someone produced a pencil and a sheet of paper.

'Fuck' was the first word suggested. Someone added 'bastard' and another boy wrote down 'shit' and then 'bollix'. 'Whore' was an acclaimed addition, as were 'bitch' and 'prick'. A boy said that we should include 'maggot' because that was what his father called him, but after a brief argument 'maggot' was dropped for not being bad enough.

The list making stopped when a small squat Christian Brother nicknamed Waddy came up behind us and, unnoticed, leaned into our circle to remove the list of bad words from a boy's hand. Brother Waddy read the list but took no action. He simply pocketed the sheet of paper and strolled away across the schoolyard with a vacant look on his face.

At the end of the day Dad gave me a lift home. I sat in the front seat of his Triumph Herald and waited for him to say something. For most of the journey home Dad hummed to himself. At one stage we had a chat about soccer. Dad told me that he had once seen the great Dixie Dean playing for Sligo against Dundalk. The way Dad remembered it, Dean had done nothing for eighty-five minutes of the match. With Sligo a goal down and no sign of anything special from Dixie, the crowd had decided that he was a has-been. People had been heading for exits when he had come to life. In the last few minutes, Dixie had moved twice. Wham, bang, two goals went in – Sligo won 2–1. It just went to show that you had to hang in there until the end if you wanted to succeed. It was just like theatre. Nothing seemed to be happening for ages and then there was that moment of brilliance that you would remember all your life.

He didn't mention that morning's rehearsals.

At home, Mother praised me for my acting. Dad told her I was going to make a first-class Roman soldier. He was sorry that he hadn't promoted me to centurion.

It was hard to know what to think. Mother hadn't seen me act and Dad had ignored me throughout except for telling me to keep a menacing look on my face. Maybe he had seen something in me. Perhaps he expected that I would go on stage one day to deliver a 'moment of brilliance' that people would remember all their lives.

The production moved smoothly after that. The dress rehearsal was uneventful and the first night deemed a resounding success.

Nobody mucked up an exit or missed a cue.

Nobody mentioned the bad-language incident.

Nobody noticed the Roman soldier's menacing look.

★

The Christian Brothers who taught in Coláiste Mhuire were big into pageants and plays that celebrated Catholicism or Ireland's glorious history of getting stuffed by the Brits – or preferably both. The lay teachers pretty much went along with whatever the Brothers wanted, but they rarely had any direct involvement in the plays.

The pageants were under the command of Brother

Matthew, a friend of my father. Dad was always hired to direct and write the pageants and, as the oldest son of Tomás Mac Anna of the Abbey Theatre, it stood to reason that I could act.

My role as a Roman soldier was my first experience as an actor. It was OK. I enjoyed getting off lessons and the backstage swordfights were great gas.

After the first pageant some of the other kids had received praise and rewards for their efforts. The guy who had played Mary, Mother of Jesus, was given a book token. People just took it for granted that I enjoyed acting. It was in my blood. How could I not?

I wasn't sure. I was shy. I didn't like fuss or being singled out. I liked having a father who was famous. I liked the sort of semi-outlaw status of coming from a theatrical family. I took it for granted that everyone went to first nights in the Abbey.

I had been dragged along by my parents to attend first nights of plays in the Abbey, the Peacock, the Eblana, the Damer, the Gate and other places. At age ten I had already sat through *A Long Day's Journey into Night* – four of the longest hours of my life, where my legs had died and my bottom had turned to marble. Afterwards Mother had told me that I was lucky to have witnessed the greatest production of that play in history. I would remember it for ever.

To me, theatre was a boring waste of my young time.

But I daren't tell that to my parents. Theatre was their religion and their passion. I don't know what they would have done if I had refused to act in a pageant or attend a first night. That said, this acting lark had potential. It got you off lessons and it increased your stature with other kids. The really great thing about acting on stage was that you didn't have to sit in the audience and get bored.

*

The next year the Brothers cast me again and once more Dad was the director.

This time my role was as a swordsman of the Fianna, Finn McCool's mythical warriors. I carried a shield and a short sword, but I had no dialogue. My job was to wave the sword in the air whenever Finn McCool ended a speech.

Dad didn't curse once during these rehearsals – everything went smoothly. I began to enjoy it. It was fun, like being in a gladiator movie.

Then the costumes arrived.

Warriors of Na Fianna had to wear silver kilts that looked like miniskirts. We were handed chain vests that had been shrunk and sprayed with gold paint. Finn McCool wore an old Irish dancing kilt and a purple blanket with a Celtic design on it. We used wooden sticks as swords and our shields were old dustbin lids painted orange.

The Brothers got into a big flap about the first night – the President of Ireland was coming. This was a wonderful opportunity to show off the school.

Eamon de Valera, President of Ireland and hero of 1916, sat in the front row, surrounded by bodyguards. There had been some kind of a threat on his life and the bodyguards were jumpy.

The production went well until the interval. For the second act, we warriors of the Fianna lined up across the stage like an honour guard. It was supposed to be a tribute to the president. An tUachtaráin Eamon de Valera stared at us blankly through small darkened glasses while we held our swords and shields high. We were supposed to maintain this noble posture until the curtains drew apart, announcing the beginning of the second act.

Just before the curtains parted, an object dropped from above, missing the president's head by inches. The bodyguards leapt from their seats and aimed their pistols at the box overhead.

In their sights was my father, who had accidentally dropped his pipe out the window of the flying-saucer lighting box in the ceiling. Dad calmly leaned out the window with his arm extended and asked, 'Can I have my pipe back, please?'

★

Hollywood came to the Abbey to make a film about the life of Sean O'Casey, though the hero was given a new name – Johnny Cassidy. This may have been because of a row with the famous Irish playwright or it could have been because an Australian actor, Rod Taylor, was playing the lead. Whatever the reason, the film, which was supposed to have been called *Young O'Casey*, was now renamed *Young Cassidy*.

I was among six boys who were given time off school to appear as extras in the film. I was the only one from my class to get picked. The others were at least a year older but I didn't mind. I was going to be in a movie. My acting career was picking up.

We played Dublin street urchins and wore shabby clothes and cloth caps. We were positioned on the street outside some false shop fronts and made to rehearse running away over and over on the command 'Action'.

After countless rehearsals a tall man singled me out. He handed me a stone and told me that I was to wait for 'action' and then hurl the stone through an enormous window. After that I was to leg it with the others. The window was truly enormous. I was only five feet away. I couldn't miss.

On the first take I threw the stone over the roof of the shop front. On the second I hit a wall. The third throw landed at the director's feet, which was good going considering that he was sitting directly behind me.

The stone was taken from me and given to a boy called Anto. On 'Action', Anto threw the stone through the enormous window and we all ran for it. They got it, first take. The tall man clapped Anto on the back.

Afterwards I felt humiliated and useless. I sat next to Anto at lunch. 'One take, one shot,' he said. He said it at regular intervals throughout the afternoon. 'One take, one shot.' Sometimes he varied it. 'One shot, one take.' He told me that he was getting paid extra for smashing the window.

I couldn't say anything because Anto was bigger and older and he could throw stones better than I could, and get paid for it.

This acting business was actually a lot harder that it looked.

The next morning, Dad brought me into the Abbey. He said that I would get a chance to watch Hollywood in action. He sat me upstairs in the balcony of the theatre and told me to stay quiet. The cast and crew were downstairs setting up.

I watched endless rehearsals of Rod Taylor saying goodbye to Maggie Smith. The scene was straightforward. Rod asked Maggie to stay with him. She replied that she could not. Then Maggie walked away from him. Rod reached out for Maggie. Maggie exited. Rod looked sad.

They did it over and over again. Each time they performed the same actions, repeated the same lines with the same intonations and adopted the same expressions.

Upstairs, I was bored rigid.

If it took this long to film a simple scene, how long did it take to film a shootout in a cowboy film or a car chase? Filming *The Man from UNCLE* must take years. It was enough to put you off films for life.

Then suddenly it was over. The actors left. The film equipment and other gear was knocked down and removed at a great pace. The theatre was clear within minutes.

I sat in the balcony alone for a while, then I wandered about. The theatre appeared empty. I opened the doors and wandered out into the lobby. Nobody knew where Dad was. I sat downstairs under a painting of Yeats and waited.

After a long time, Dad emerged from somewhere to take me home. 'Well, now you've seen how movies are made,' Dad said. "That's something you'll never forget.'

★

I was eleven when I met Pádraig Pearse. Pádraig was tall, skinny and slightly confused. He wore a flabby green uniform, two gun belts and a wide-rimmed khaki hat that made him look like an Irish Pancho Villa.

This Pearse did not come across as the kind of guy who could lead the Irish nation to freedom. He didn't look as though he'd be much use to the Mexicans either.

But when the spotlights came on and the imitation Pádraig Pearse strolled out into the centre of Croke Park, he inspired just as much turmoil and bloodshed in the name of Mother Ireland as the original. The difference was that these heroics were part of 'Aiséirí', the special Glóirreim celebrations of 1966 to mark the fiftieth anniversary of the Easter Rising. It was only make-believe.

A bunch from my school was picked as extras for the crowd scenes. Most were picked because they acted in the school plays, others because they lived near Croke Park. Once again, I got the gig because my father was directing.

After an hour of rehearsals, some of us were picked out for more important tasks – I was promoted to letter-carrier. My job was to walk on at the end holding up a massive plastic letter *E*. This formed the final letter of ÉIRE, the visual centrepiece of the closing celebrations of the birth of the new republic spawned by the Rising.

It was a massive production. The entire Irish army seemed to have been divided up as either insurrectionists, British army or civilians. The civilians got the worst of it. Every time there was a riot scene, the soldiers charged the crowd and chased them out of the stadium. For some reason, the audience always cheered whenever the crowd got hammered.

Some of the soldiers used the battle scenes to settle a few old scores. People said there were more casualties in the dressing rooms after each show than during the whole of 1916.

It should have been a humdinger. There was action, spectacle, colour, excitement and schmaltz – everything you could possibly ask for in a decent epic. But the four-night run coincided with the worst storm to hit Dublin for decades. Speeches were distorted. Actors were blown off their feet. Props ended up in the stands.

One night a gust of wind totally demolished a British armoured car. It was hard for an army to maintain credibility when its heavy artillery was floating somewhere over Hill 16.

On the third night the wind snapped off the bottom half of my letter. From the stands it appeared that the glorious, heroic blood sacrifice of 1916 had culminated in the birth of the new republic of ÉIRF. Diehard nationalists must have been mortified.

RTÉ also chose that week to show *Insurrection*, their rival big-budget account of the 1916 Rising. Modern technology now brought Pádraig Pearse into the living rooms of the people of Ireland. Croke Park in the middle of the hurricane season was no competition.

Because of the freak weather, 'Aiséirí: Gloírreim na Casca' drew poor crowds for the first two nights – insurrectionists sometimes outnumbered the audience by three to one – but the show received a lot of acclaim and finished its run to full houses. It was deemed to have been an artistic triumph, which meant that it lost a packet.

As far as we were concerned, the only important thing was that the letter-carriers be paid. We made representations to management. There were some frank discussions. At one stage there was talk of a strike – there would be no new nation at the end of the show, we warned, unless financial terms were agreed.

I appealed to my father. He told me to hang on. Something good was coming.

Eventually, we were instructed to wait until the last night, when each letter-carrier would receive a special surprise.

On the final night everyone was handed a brown envelope with a newly minted, limited-edition, souvenir ten-shilling piece inside. One side of the silver coin showed Pearse's profile, while the reverse featured an illustration of *An Cliabh Solais* (The Sword of Light).

It wasn't exactly what we had in mind.

But the real surprise was that we couldn't spend them. The coin would be extremely important many years from now, people told us. We'd appreciate it when we were grown up. We would show it to our grandchildren. 'Bollix to my grandchildren,' a boy said. 'I want to go and buy things.'

None of the adults would listen. The way they looked at it, we had been paid for our labour with coins of inestimable historical and social significance. We were told that Pearse himself would have approved. That was the start of my disillusionment with Pearse.

The final night's wrap party was the scene of much intense coin dealing. Some of the letter-carriers sold their Pearse coins to disgruntled adults at half-price and went off to buy Cokes and sweets. A half-cut sergeant bought one for a pound. It was the bargain of the century, he boasted – his grandchildren would know where he had been during Easter 1966.

But I held on to mine. I felt guilty because of all the school lectures I remembered about the suffering and sacrifice of the martyrs of 1916.

A week afterwards my mother informed me that we were related to Seán Mac Diarmada, one of the original signatories of the 1916 Proclamation. Now it would be blasphemous to spend the ten-bob bit. The coin was more than a souvenir, it was a symbol of nationhood.

For weeks I kept the coin in a small plastic pouch in a matchbox in my pocket, as you would a pet mouse. At school I showed it to my friends. Some were impressed. A few were jealous. All laughed when they found out that I wasn't allowed to spend it.

I discovered that being related to Seán Mac Diarmada was no big deal either. One of the guys in my class boasted that his mother was a daughter of James Connolly and his father a brother-in-law of Pearse himself. 'Mac Diarmada was small fry,' he said.

That lunchtime I fought that classmate until both of us were bleeding. The feud continued at break times each day for a week. Finally a Christian Brother put a halt to it and then gave both of us four across the palms with the leather strap for fighting in the yard.

Gradually the power of the special coin waned. Pearse just didn't seem that important anymore. Most kids I knew were far more interested in the next Manchester United game or the latest from The Beatles or who had the biggest collection of sixty-four-page comics. Nobody seemed to give two hoots about the 1916 Rising.

Besides, the Christian Brothers loved Pearse and anyone the Brothers liked must be a wimp.

One day I walked into the Candy Shop around the corner from the school and swapped my 1916-special-souvenir-Pádraig-Pearse coin for ten sixty-four-page comics, that week's editions of the *Victor* and the *Valiant*, a box of Aero chocolate bars and a plastic German paratrooper's helmet.

For years afterwards, I felt like a traitor.

★

The Abbey Theatre had a huge success with *Borstal Boy*, adapted from the memoir by Brendan Behan. The play was a hit at home, but it was also successful worldwide. Dad directed it on Broadway in 1970 and the show won a Tony for best new play. The Tony Award was placed on our mantelpiece at home.

Borstal Boy was invited to Paris for a short run. They needed a couple of young lads to play various roles and I was cast in two small parts – as a newspaper boy and a snobby altar boy. I didn't know if I liked the play or not – it was difficult to decide. When you are close to something it's always difficult to know exactly how to feel about it. Dennis, whose father had adapted the book into a play, was also cast in several small roles, including that of a newspaper boy.

We played for a short run in Dublin. The play began in total darkness and then a flash bomb went off on stage. My job was to run on soon afterwards waving newspapers and shouting out headlines such as 'Bomb in Liverpool' and 'Read all about it'. Dennis did exactly the same thing coming from the other side of the stage. Each of us wore giant sandwich boards, which were awkward to put on and which made walking difficult.

In the second act I played a snobby altar boy. I had to walk across the stage to the centre, observe a group of shabby-looking borstal boys and walk past them quickly with my nose in the air. People said I was a terrific snobby altar boy, but I got the feeling that at least some of them were only saying that because I was the director's son.

We played the Abbey for a couple of weeks without incident. I enjoyed being on stage. I loved the sense of the audience out there in the seats. I could feel them, but I daren't look at them. It was thrilling being part of a big production. I figured that I could get used to this kind of life. I might never have to go back to school. I liked the idea that I could tour the world performing in plays.

The company flew to Paris. I received a lot of attention and praise from the actors and crew. My father's secretary was very sweet to me.

We played at a theatre named the Michelet-Odeon. On the first night the Duke and Duchess of Argyle were in the audience. We were all invited up to their suite in a posh hotel afterwards for drinks.

The duchess was in her fifties, but she was still extremely beautiful. She wore a diamond pendant around her neck. She had an extraordinary effect on the male actors, many of whom surrounded her and competed to light her cigarettes and fetch her drinks.

She spent some time with me. She put her hand on my head and told me to keep up the acting. The smell of her perfume was pleasant, almost intoxicating. I thought she was wonderful.

A middle-aged actor sat on the edge of the duke's seat. He asked the duke what he was supposed to call him. He had never met royalty before, he said. The duke politely replied that the actor could call him Ian.

The actor thought that this was extraordinary. He said that if he wasn't sitting there on the edge of the duke's chair he would never had thought that such a thing was possible. 'Call me Bill,' he told the duke.

Bill spent the rest of the night telling Ian about his life in the theatre. The duke remained polite, but he looked thoroughly bored. He looked like he wanted to toss Bill out the window.

I discovered a small café across the road from the hotel where a girl named Lisa worked behind the counter. I had learned that the French for pineapple juice was *ananas* and most days I went into the bar and ordered *ananas*. Although I enjoyed the pineapple juice, I was really there because I had fallen in love with Lisa, who was dark and beautiful and wore her hair in a pageboy fringe. She was at least four years older than me and ignored me completely.

One day an Abbey stagehand with whom I had struck up a casual acquaintanceship came into the bar and joined me at the counter. He ordered a beer and bought me an *ananas*. Somehow the stagehand managed to put together enough French to ask Lisa out.

That night and every night for the remainder of the run, the stagehand appeared at my side just before curtain up to boast about what he and Lisa had gotten up during the previous evening's date. I understood very little of the intimate details, but his bragging broke my fourteen-year-old heart all the same. It also destroyed my image of Lisa as the beautiful and perfect French girl. Now I figured that if she went out with that eejit she must be a bit of an eejit herself and I gave up going for to the small café for *ananas*.

The experience made me wish I was older, if only so that I could understand what the stagehand had been talking about.

★

Dad brought Mom with him to Paris. In the daytime, I spent a lot of time walking around the city with my parents (my brothers and sisters were being minded in Howth by a stern little woman from Limerick hired by my parents). My parents had struck up a friendship with Guy, a Parisian who seemed to have a perfect, permanent suntan. He was a jovial man who took his role as our personal tour guide very seriously.

He took us to Place de la Concorde and Versailles, but he also showed us around areas of the city where incidents had taken place during the Second World War. My father filmed everything with his Bell & Howell hand-held 8mm. Guy wore a tragic expression whenever Dad filmed him at the location of a sad incident.

Guy was a schoolteacher with a family of his own, though he

never brought them to meet us. One day he asked permission to take me to his school to talk to the pupils about Howth and Irish life. I was around the same age as his students and it would be good for them to hear from a boy from a different country and culture. Dad said OK.

Guy collected me from the theatre one morning and drove me to his school on the outskirts of Paris. He hung a map of Ireland on the blackboard and asked me to indicate the location of Howth and tell the pupils all about my life in Ireland. I did my best. I wasn't great at geography, but I managed to find Howth and drew a chalk circle around it. Everything was going fine until one of the pupils set fire to a ball of paper and threw it at the dustbin near the blackboard. 'Do they have the fire brigades in Ireland?' the boy asked.

Guy got angry and shouted at them in French before putting out the fire in the bin with a glass of water from a tap at the back of the room. Most of the students ignored him. One threw a rolled up paper at me. I threw it back. I was beginning to enjoy this class. Guy, however, was disgruntled that I had chosen to lark about when I should have been talking about Ireland. The session on life in Ireland was abandoned. Guy placed me outside the classroom on a chair while the class resumed normal lessons.

At lunchtime Guy brought me home to meet his family. On the drive over, he told me that his wife had been going to give him 'the divorce' but that they had made up and all was OK.

At his apartment he left me outside while he went in to tell his wife that there would be a guest for lunch. He was gone for a long time. Then he reappeared and beckoned me to follow him.

His wife and kids sat at a small round table. They looked surprised to see Guy, but totally shocked to see me. His eldest daughter kept staring at me through strong glasses that made her look permanently astounded – as though they all thought I was Guy's Irish love child. Little was said after the initial introductions. We ate a silent lunch, after which Guy dropped me back to the theatre.

I don't know why Guy took me back to his apartment. At the time it had seemed like a perfectly natural thing to do. Perhaps I was used to not questioning the odd behaviour of my parents' friends.

That night Dad asked me how the day had gone and I told him that I had talked to Guy's class and that one of the kids had set fire to a ball of paper and thrown it. I said that I'd gone to have lunch with Guy's family but that the experience had been weird. 'Good, good,' said Dad, absentmindedly. 'Well done, Ferdia. I'm glad you're enjoying Paris.'

On the last night of *Borstal Boy* in Paris, the flash bomb failed to go off. Everyone stood around in pitch blackness for an age. Finally someone poked me and told me to go on.

I walked out into the centre of the stage, yelling out my lines. From the other side Dennis came on, also yelling.

When the flash bomb went off we both jumped in the air. I lost my cloth cap and the sandwich board slipped. I made it to the far side before everything fell – newspapers, sandwich board and my braces, which had snapped. Later people said it looked extremely convincing, as though a bomb had been set off in order to bump off the newspaper boys.

I returned from Paris as a veteran Abbey theatre player. I was confident that my acting career had taken off and I looked forward to the next school play – there would probably be another movie soon. Acting was a good gig. I told my father that the next time he directed a school play I wanted dialogue.

＊

When we got back from Paris I thought we would never see Guy again.

I was wrong.

In October, he came to Howth. At first Dad and Mom welcomed him and showed him around. Dad disappeared into the city to direct a new play at the Abbey, so the rest of us had to look after Guy.

He was supposed to stay for a weekend, but the weekend turned into a week and then the week became a fortnight. He got upset if he didn't get his own way. He liked to lock himself into the bathroom for hours and expected to be waited on all the time. He kept reminding us of the great time he had shown us in Paris. 'I brought the boy home to my apartment for lunch,' he said.

One day I found Mother really upset in the kitchen. She told me that Guy was driving her mad. She wanted to write him a filthy, nasty letter.

I was intrigued. 'What's a filthy, nasty letter?' I asked. Mother explained that it was the kind of letter you wrote to a person when you wanted to tell what you really thought of them. 'You don't mince your words,' she said. Before adding, 'That man is too much.'

To please my mother I sat down at the front doorstep with a pen and paper and wrote Guy a filthy, nasty letter. Mother had explained that you didn't mince your words, which meant that you used as many bad words as you knew. I opened with 'Guy you bastard', and went on from there.

When I was finished I was delighted with myself. I had done something that would please Mother. I showed her the letter – she read the first few lines and screamed before sending me to my room. 'I can't deal with this now,' she said.

When Dad came home Mom showed him my filthy, nasty letter. Dad came to my room to see me. 'There was no need for that kind of thing,' he said. He told me that he had no idea that I knew so many foul words. 'I hope you didn't get it from me.'

Guy always had a superb suntan. In the winter light he sometimes looked as though he was glowing with health and vitality and energy.

He also looked as though he was never going to leave. Then one day my sister discovered his suntan spray and decided to give herself an all-over tan. Emerging from the bathroom after an hour, she looked as though she had just flown in from St Tropez. Guy's eyes nearly popped out. For some reason, the discovery of his permanent suntan spray greatly distressed him.

He wore a sad face and went home the next morning. My sister's St Tropez tan faded a few days later.

★

That year's school pageant focused on the story of Noah's Ark. I played Japheth, one of Noah's sons. I had several lines as well as a small speech at the end. The speech was crucial to the message of the pageant. After the flood Japheth was given a vision of heaven by the Almighty. He was to report this vision to his father, Noah, and tell him of the riches and rewards that lay in store for all true believers. Japheth gave a roll call of all the Irish heroes he saw in heaven, amongst them Finn McCool, Cúchulain, Michael Collins, James Connolly and Brian Boru.

Rehearsals went extremely well. My confidence soared. This time I didn't even mind my costume – a strange-looking sack that appeared to have had dried seaweed stitched onto the front in the shape of a Celtic cross.

The first night went smoothly until it came to my big

speech. I froze. I couldn't remember any of the lines except for the one about heaven. So I pointed into the audience as I had been directed and tried to name all the famous Irish heroes I saw seated beside Our Lord. Nothing came. I stood like a zombie with my finger pointed at somebody's mother in the second row. Other boys tried to prompt me, but I couldn't hear them. I could hear the front rows squirming in their seats and I could hear coughs and whispers.

Finally, I named the names of the heroes of heaven. Mussolini was the first. There was a huge gasp from the audience but, unable to stop myself and not knowing what I was saying except that I had managed to finally remember the names of some famous people, I went on – James Bond, Taras Bulba and Genghis Khan… I may have added Rasputin and Stalin to the company, I can't remember. I'm nearly positive that I didn't say Hitler.

I ran out of names and stopped.

Immediately, I became aware of a profound silence in the auditorium. Beside me I could hear my fellow actors sniggering. None of them could say their lines for giggling. Somehow one of the boys got it together and said a line of dialogue. The others sorted themselves out and the pageant concluded.

Backstage, the sense of shock was etched on the face of every Christian Brother. One of their pupils had just announced to the assembled mass of parents that, amongst other villains, Benito Mussolini was to be found in heaven. Their system of education had been indicted by one of their own pupils.

I was taken aside by a Brother and asked what I thought I was doing.

I said that I was sorry but that I had forgotten my lines and that those names were the only ones I could think of. He asked me what books I had been reading. I didn't know what to say.

In the end he couldn't do much to the son of the director of the pageant so he left me alone.

We all went back onstage for the curtain call. The rows of smiles from the audience seemed brighter than all the spotlights in the place. The 'Mussolini incident' was never mentioned again. Well, not by an adult anyway. My father behaved as though nothing untoward had happened on stage. Maybe it was his way of saying, I'll forget about Mussolini if you forget about the time I said 'fuck' into the microphone.

The next day I retired from acting. I just wasn't cut out for it.

6

Off the Coast of Dad

The president of America had an orange face.

JFK had the weirdest suntan I had ever seen or else he had dyed his face and hands. I saw him for a few seconds on O'Connell Street as he swung past in his open-topped car. He looked powerful and noble and yet oddly, conspicuously carrot-coloured.

I was eight when my father brought me to see JFK. I knew that John Wayne was American, along with cowboys and peanut butter. I was aware that the US had won the Second World War, but that was about the extent of my knowledge of the country. I didn't see why I had to be dragged into the city to see some boring old president. It would have been different if we had been going to see John Wayne.

I had no interest in the American president, but I was glad to be spending time with my dad. This was the first thing we had done together, or at least the first that I can remember apart from the time we queued for hours in the cold to see *The Longest Day* at the Ambassador. He was away a lot in my early childhood – the theatre, lecturing, adjudicating – things kept him away from home, so I relished the time I spent with him.

There was a huge crowd on O'Connell Street and it took us ages to find a good vantage point along the route. There were too many people milling about and I couldn't see anything except the backs of coats, so Dad lifted me high and sat me on his shoulders.

I towered above an ocean of happy, smiling faces. What seemed like a million people lined both sides of the street. Heads jutted out of windows. I saw figures peering from rooftops. The crowd waved streamers and flags even though there was no sign of the presidential motorcade. The excitement of the crowd intrigued me.

Finally, a bunch of motorcycle cops sailed into O'Connell Street from the direction of the Ambassador Cinema. In a moment, a sleek, black, open-topped car swung into view bearing a blond man who was smiling a blazing-white smile and waving. JFK beamed down at us for a slow-motion moment. His chiselled, handsome face stood out clearly, perhaps because he was the first extremely tanned man I had ever seen. He seemed friendly. The crowd erupted all around me as thousands of hands waved back as though waving to the President of the World. By the time I waved too, JFK had whipped past and was gone.

And that was it.

I wasn't sure what all the fuss had been about. We had gone to all that effort for just one glimpse of an orangey man waving from a moving car. It didn't make any sense to me. I would rather have seen a movie or played soccer in the front garden.

A few months later I was watching TV one evening when the programme was interrupted by a news flash about Kennedy's assassination. The president had been shot in Dallas.

I went into the kitchen to tell my parents, but they didn't believe me. They thought that I had been watching a movie about the Second World War. Kennedy had fought in the war, he'd been wounded, Dad told me. That must have been what I had heard.

'He's not wounded, he's assassinated,' I said, but they still didn't believe me so I went back to the TV.

Later, when the news was confirmed, my parents were shocked. We watched television together. The president had been picked off by a sniper while travelling through Dallas in an open car in a procession just like the one Dad and me had seen on O'Connell Street. Texas governor John Connolly, who was sitting beside JFK had been wounded and survived while the president had died.

I asked Dad why the president couldn't have just been winged too. 'Why did the Americans shoot their own president?'

'These things happen,' Dad said.

*

My dad's face was bigger than other dads' faces. Whenever I dropped in to his office at the Abbey to collect lunch money or to get a lift home, I noticed that Dad was taller than most people and that his face appeared larger.

I got used to finding him hunched up in an uncomfortable front-row seat in the Abbey or the Peacock directing rehearsals. Sometimes he was upstairs in the Abbey's rehearsal space, balancing precariously on a rickety chair. To drive he had to cram himself into his car as though he had been inserted into his seat with a giant shoehorn.

He had a funny way of walking sometimes, head down and both arms going like pistons. Whenever he stood still for a moment and drew himself up to his full height, he seemed to dwarf everyone around him.

At home in the bungalow in Howth he sat in his black leather easy chair in the front room, which we called Dad's Study. The chair squeaked and the footrest sprang up from underneath like a secret weapon whenever he leaned back. We thought the *yang* noise the footrest made was hilarious.

When we were bold he turned that big stern face on us, sometimes with his cheeks puffed out like he was about to blow us through the wall.

When we were good he smiled at us. If we were competing to get his attention by trying to amuse him, he laughed and his face lit up like a statue coming to life. It was reassuring to have that big face beaming down upon you.

The world came to him when he sat in that chair. He watched TV while reading scripts and making notes. He placed miniature stage sets complete with tiny chairs and tables and sometimes mini cardboard figures on his knees while he charted lighting changes and stage movements. Sometimes he worked while The Beatles or Joan Baez or Maria Callas or Broadway music played on the gramophone. He usually had a book or a script open on his lap as he watched the news on TV, with his dinner on the small table in front of him and his kids around him like fallen leaves.

He smoked cigarettes constantly. This amounted to him sticking a lit fag in his mouth and leaving it there to build up into a leaning pillar of ash. Once the ash toppled onto his lapel, he brushed it off. Then he lit another fag and the process started over. I don't think he ever inhaled.

Dad dressed like an eccentric bohemian – he wore cravats and waistcoats. Sometimes he wore cardigans. His primary colours were dark or navy, but he always added a dash of red or light blue in the cravats he wore or in the handkerchiefs that he stuck in his top pocket. I never saw him wear a tie. For a time he wore a Russian winter hat that made him look like a Cossack. When he left the house to go to work he didn't look as though he was going to a job in an office.

★

When I was nine my father took a position as a guest director with the National Theatre of Iceland. The family accompanied him to live in Reykjavik, where we stayed for a year.

The trip over was my first time on a plane. I remember that the engines were loud and the ascent hurt my ears until the Aer Lingus hostess gave us boiled sweets. It was impossible to get comfortable on the seats.

We lived in an apartment on a snow-covered street. Iceland seemed much the same as Ireland except that there was snow most of the time and the potatoes were blue when you cut into them. I liked the snow, but refused to have anything to do with blue potatoes.

Our apartment had an intercom, the first we had ever seen. My sister and I were really taken by the thing, but our little brother absolutely adored playing with it. We had great gas taking it in turns to go outside to ring the buzzer and then engaging in mad dialogue across the intercom. The voices on the intercom sounded like crazy space aliens.

To put a stop to this carry-on, Dad told us that there was a vicious, scary demon in Reykjavik called the Black Baboo. The Black Baboo preyed on kids. It was best not to go outdoors without being accompanied by an adult. I didn't buy the Black Baboo business at all, but my little brother Niall was intimidated by thoughts of a scary demon that was waiting for the chance to carry off little Irish kids.

However, Niall still liked to be the first to run to the intercom. Standing on a chair to reach the speaker, he always answered cheerfully. 'Will I let you in?' He often pressed the door-release button without waiting to find out who was outside.

One day I snuck outside and pressed the bell to our apartment. Niall answered as usual. 'Will I let you in?'

I put on a deep, scary voice. 'This is the Black Babooooo.'

I heard a scream and a *clunk* as the intercom phone hit the wall, then silence.

I waited outside for a long time before anyone would let me back in. My parents were furious with me – Niall sat in a corner completely pale. The prank had worked too well. Dad took me aside for a long lecture. He was really angry. He had not brought me all the way to Iceland just so that I could play wicked tricks on my little brother. The Black Baboo was never to be mentioned again.

The first play Dad directed was *Romeo and Juliet* and I was allowed to sit in the front row to watch the rehearsals. The play was OK. I still found theatre dull, and I wasn't much interested in the lovey-dovey stuff between Romeo and Juliet. However, I really enjoyed the swordfights. They were the only things in the play that weren't in Icelandic.

The Icelandic government had provided Dad with an official translator, though his presence was unnecessary because all the actors spoke fluent English. Nevertheless, this was the National Theatre of Iceland, the play was in Icelandic and all theatre business had to be conducted through the official language of the country, so a translator was to hand at all times. Dad gave directions and the actors carried them out. A few seconds later the official translator translated Dad's instructions into Icelandic.

After a time, as he realised that his input was being ignored, the official translator's voice dropped lower and then lower still. Within an hour the official translator looked like a forlorn individual. He sat alone, apparently whispering to himself.

I was very impressed that my father was in charge of so many people and that he had been given his own translator. I still didn't care for the theatre. Going to plays seemed more a duty than a passion. It struck me as something that people thought they needed to do and I swore that when I grew up I wasn't going to bother with plays.

I went to school at the American Embassy facility. I sat at my own desk in a small classroom with several American kids, three boys and two girls as well as a slightly older girl who must have been around twelve or thirteen. The older girl was named Ally and she was Icelandic-American. Ally took a shine to me and looked out for me.

Everyone thought it was hilarious when I told them that there were fifty kids to a class in primary school in Ireland. They also thought it was funny that kids sat two to a desk. I didn't mention the leather strap or the bamboo cane. I didn't want them to think that we were total savages.

In the embassy school there was no leather, no bamboo cane and no corporal punishment of any kind. If you messed up in class, you were assigned punishment lines. You had to write fifty lines for getting a sum wrong and more if you were caught talking or messing about when you should have been paying attention. The teachers insisted that all handwriting should be neat and legible.

They also placed a big emphasis on Greek mythology, where there was a lot of stuff about heads getting severed and people getting changed into animals by magic. I liked the all-powerful Zeus, who always seemed to be losing his rag and wreaking hideous vengeance on mortals. I was terrified of Medusa, with her hair of snakes and her look that would turn a person to stone. One of my favourites was the story of the Minotaur. I liked the way the creature looked in the illustrations. I thought that Heracles was a more impressive and believable superhero than Superman, who always struck me as too perfect and essentially a bit of a swot at heart. I felt anguish at the story of Icarus who flew so close to the sun that the wax on his wings melted, plunging him to his doom. I read and re-read the story, hoping that I had missed the bit where he survived the fall. I loved the exotic, slightly scary names as well as the graphic and frequently savage illustrations in the book of Greek myths. I wondered why they didn't teach this stuff in Coláiste Mhuire.

I didn't get on with the American kids.

At lunchtime they challenged each other to dares. They climbed high walls and hung from the railing by their ankles and pulled other stunts that I didn't want to do. They liked to compete with each other and had a different style of playing than the kids at home. They weren't friendly and that didn't help my shyness.

I hung around with Ally. She hated school and didn't want to be stuck in Iceland for the rest of her life. She wanted to visit other places, but first she needed to go back and live in the sunny US. She was tired of wearing thick woollen sweaters all the time.

For lunch one day we were served spinach soup. It was green and looked disgusting, but Popeye ate spinach so it must be good. I tried a spoonful and hated it. I asked the canteen lady if I could have something else instead. The canteen lady was fair haired and patient and wore a kindly smile. She told me that spinach soup was good for me. I still wouldn't eat the soup. 'I'm very disappointed,' the lady smiled.

It turned out that the canteen lady was also the school librarian, the post mistress and the person in charge of stores.

She was also a compete wagon.

From then on she made sure that I had spinach for lunch almost every day. When I complained that none of the other kids had been given spinach, the lady put on her reasonable voice and explained that the other kids always ate their spinach when they were given it. I was the only one who had let the side down. She gave me spinach with fish, spinach with meat, spinach with pasta and spinach sandwiches – I continued to refuse to eat the stuff. Even when my friend Ally attempted to intervene, the canteen lady continued to act oh so reasonably and do exactly as she pleased. I went hungry a lot.

I plucked up the courage to tell Dad about the spinach situation. He said that he would have a word. The next morning he came into the school with me and went to see the canteen lady.

That lunchtime I got a cheese sandwich.

The next day everyone – including me – got spinach soup.

For the rest of the school term, Spinach Woman ruled all.

Everyone in Iceland was tall and blue eyed and good looking. The actors and actresses from the National Theatre of Iceland, who frequently dropped by to visit us at home, were the tallest and best looking of all. My mom and dad often threw parties at our apartment to celebrate first nights – the Icelanders loved parties. There were no bars in the country and alcohol was banned, so people drank a kind of homebrew. It was strong stuff, apparently, and actors and writers and other theatre personnel got absolutely legless in our apartment several times and had to sleep on the floor or on the sofa.

There didn't seem to be any problem about the illegal hootch. In the sixties Iceland had no police force except for a couple of traffic cops. There was no need because Iceland had no murders or muggings and burglaries were virtually unknown. Nobody in authority was going to get too distressed about illegal booze.

There was one thing that I couldn't figure out, though. The married couples amongst the actors seemed to swap partners every time I saw them. No husband ever seemed to have the same wife more than a couple of times. At one party in our house after the first night of *Romeo*, an actor introduced me to his 'wife' and later to his 'girlfriend' – and the 'wife' and the 'girlfriend' seemed to get along fine. Later, the 'wife' went home with her 'boyfriend'.

I couldn't understand how a person could be married to someone and then show up with a completely different person a short time later. I didn't understand how a man could have a wife as well as a girlfriend. I asked Dad about it. He told me that Icelanders were extremely open-minded people. They were not like married couples in Ireland. 'Blame the Vikings,' Dad said. 'They started it.'

Dad's explanation baffled me, but I knew enough to give up asking. I decided that it was impossible to figure out grown-ups. Every time I thought I had learned about adult behaviour, some eejit went and changed the rules.

One day Dad took us to visit the American Air Force base in Reykjavik, but the authorities wouldn't let us in. 'Security concerns,' an officer said. Dad was disappointed. Like us, he wanted to see the rockets. Later Dad's friend, the writer Halldor Laxness, told us that nearly all Icelanders resented the presence of an American military base in their country. He said that the least the Americans could do was to offer people free tours of the place.

To make up for the disappointment, Dad brought us to the movies instead to see a British comedy called *Make Mine Mink*. Later he took us swimming in an indoor-pool facility that had been built near one of Iceland's hot springs, to make use of the natural hot waters. *Make Mine Mink* seemed to be the only film showing in Iceland during our stay. Dad took me to see it at least three times. I got sick of the sight of Terry Thomas' moustache and the gap in his teeth.

One night the top of my middle finger was severed in an accident with a sliding door. The sliding doors belonged to a series of tall roomy wardrobes where a child could play hide and seek. Our babysitter or some kid we were playing with slammed a sliding door and I felt a sharp pain in my fingers. When I looked down the top of my middle finger was hanging by a thread of skin. There was blood everywhere. Our babysitter fainted.

Dad appeared from somewhere. Perhaps he was home all the time or maybe someone sent for him. Anyway, he draped a towel around my hand and told me to try to make sure that the top of my finger didn't fall off.

Dad drove me to the hospital, where a jolly American surgeon sewed the top of my finger back on. He told us cheerfully that the finger would probably be hideously scarred for a long time but that, if we came back to him in a couple of years, he would perform plastic surgery and make it look like new. The doctor also cautioned that the finger would hurt every time it rained. He was right. For many years my middle finger began to throb at the first hint of rain.

★

Shortly after we returned from Iceland, Dad bought a cream-coloured Triumph. One day a mechanic in the garage borrowed the car without permission to go on a moonlight spin. Instead he drove it over a cliff. Miraculously, the mechanic survived unscathed, but the car was a total write-off. At breakfast the next morning we examined the photograph of Dad's Triumph Herald in a mangled heap at the bottom of a cliff in Wicklow. I was astonished that the car we knew so well could appear in the newspaper in such a state. I kept looking at Dad to see if he was really OK – he was amused by the incident. All he said was that he was glad nobody had been hurt. He didn't mind taking the bus to work.

Within a couple of weeks Dad got a new car, a black Austin Cambridge that he kept for many years. He took me with him when he adjudicated at amateur drama festivals all over the country. It was like a town hall version of the Oscars. I bumped up and down on the red plastic seats on our way to Arklow or Athlone or Waterford or Kilkenny. I sat through endless versions of O'Casey's *Juno and the Paycock* and Synge's *Riders to the Sea* along with several versions of a musical called *Blue Moon*. Dad warned me not to fall asleep. I would disgrace him and undermine the Abbey Theatre. So I sat like a well-brought-up boy with perfect manners and got through the nights until the moment when Dad gave his summing up and awarded the winners prizes. Afterwards, the committee that had organised the festival always gave Dad a commemorative plate. At one stage there were dozens of these plates above the mantelpiece in the study, next to the photos from *Captain Lightfoot* and a framed *Proclamation of the Irish Republic*. I couldn't see any reason why anyone would want a commemorative plate with a dodgy painting on it. It was no good to look at, you couldn't eat off it and it seemed to serve no purpose unless you needed to cover up a gash in the wallpaper. But Dad seemed to like them.

Adult values made no sense at all.

On the way home from the festivals, I usually went to sleep in the back of the car. I always woke up the instant the car engine roared up the steep incline of our driveway.

Dad and me went to James Bond films too. Sometimes we went to war movies or cowboy films. Occasionally, Dad dropped me off at the cartoon cinema on Grafton Street. Once he forgot to collect me on time and I sat through endless reruns of Mickey and Minnie and Bugs and Daffy. The experience put me off Mickey Mouse for life.

Bond movies were always good, but the Matt Helm movies with Dean Martin were pretty awful. *In Like Flint* starred James Coburn, who was so skinny and smug and so dull that he made me want to root for the baddies except that the baddies seemed even sillier. Dad said that *Flint* was 'a bit daft'. He took me to *Planet of the Apes*. I was his excuse to go and see crazy escapist movies. He seemed to like the film, but he didn't say anything about it. I figured that deep down, Dad was the same movie age as me.

Dad brought home Beatles and Joan Baez albums. The albums were supposed to be for me, but he played them himself on his peculiar wooden gramophone in the study, where everything seemed to play at a slightly slower speed than normal. Even the radio announcers seemed to speak sluggishly on Dad's gramophone. But when Dad played his showbiz records everything sounded right. He favourites were 'Waiting for Jane' by Eddie 'Rochester' Anderson and 'Lullaby of Broadway' by Dick Powell. Maybe the gramophone objected to rock. Dad also played an album of cowboy songs, *How the West Was Won*. I liked the cowboy stuff better than The Beatles.

I accompanied Dad to first nights of plays in the Abbey, some of which he directed. He enjoyed them all; I hated being trapped in those uncomfortable seats. At a crap film, it was easy to get up and walk out. In a theatre I felt too intimidated to ask people in the row to let me out. There was no escape in a theatre.

One day Dad handed me *Catch-22* by Joseph Heller. A few weeks later, he gave me *Slaughterhouse Five* by Kurt Vonnegut. He encouraged me to read, but he rarely bought me books; instead he passed on the ones he liked. There were books everywhere when I was growing up. In the study books peeked out from under the tables and chairs. There were piles by the sofa and on the desk and shelves.

Once Dad came home from giving a lecture in Wales and gave me a huge poster of 'Fern Hill' by Dylan Thomas. I hung the poster on the wall of my room, where it stayed for years. I loved the last lines:

> *Time held me green and dying*
> *Though I sang in my chains like the sea.*

I didn't know what it meant exactly, but I didn't care because the words were like music. The poster hung on my bedroom wall until my late teens, when I came home drunk one night and tore 'Fern Hill' to bits.

Dad also brought home the LP of *Under Milk Wood*, the one with Richard Burton. Milk Wood was a fishing village like Howth, and even though I couldn't identify with the sailors or the drunks or the lovelorn, I loved the mad voices and I could feel the crazy rhythm of the words inside me. I played the LP constantly.

Dad may have been on a mission to introduce me to culture and entertainment, but he drew the line at discussing what we had just listened to or seen or read. It was as though the event itself was enough. Maybe he thought I needed to make up my own mind about things. Why ruin it with analysis or debate?

When I tried to get him to talk, Dad usually made a single observation and then left it at that. With the Matt Helm film *The Silencers*, for instance, Dad said that Dean Martin went to sleep after the opening titles. After four-and-a-half hours of Sergei Bondarchuk's *War and Peace*, Dad's verdict was 'brilliant, but it goes on a bit'.

I picked up on his style. When he asked me what I thought about *The Dirty Dozen*, I told him I liked the German helmets. 'Hmmmph,' he said.

One night at the Abbey I watched as a drunken man was carried out of a play by two ushers. The man seemed to be asleep. I asked Dad who he was and Dad explained that I had just seen the theatre critic from one of Ireland's most prestigious newspapers. Dad didn't think much of the critics and almost never talked about them. He was interested in the reaction of the audience, not the critics.

I once heard him criticise an academic turned bad actor as a 'twit'. He didn't think that it was wise to allow academics to have any kind of creative control in a theatre or in any artistic endeavour. However, he rarely said anything negative about the actors he worked with, even the ones who occasionally showed up for a production drunk. He liked creative people. He respected the audience. He adored the theatre. The rest didn't appear to concern him unduly.

★

I was fifteen when Dad moved out. Mother gathered us together in the study and told us in a sorrowful voice that Dad would not be returning home. She had no idea why he had decided to leave. He was living in a hotel. She said that she didn't want to talk about it because it was too painful. She wanted us to all stick together. There would be tough times ahead, but we would be fine if we loved one another. She gave me a meaningful look. She told me that I was the oldest and the new Man of the House. She was relying on me. I told her that I would look after everyone, though I had no notion of what that meant. I wanted to make Mother feel better. She gave me a warm smile and told me she knew that I would not let her or the family down.

I went to bed hating Dad. He had dumped us. How could he just walk away from us all and go to live in a hotel? What would become of us? I had no answers to the questions that were pinging about in my mind.

That weekend I took my new role as Man of the House seriously. I had to save the family; their well-being was now my responsibility. I would quit school and get a job on the fishing boats – my friend Nessan knew some of the fishermen. He would put in a word for me.

The next morning, without being asked, I went to the Summit for cigarettes and matches and bottles of stout. I asked the barman to put it on our slate.

I looked after Naoise. I didn't fight with my sisters and I was nice to my brothers.

There was no word from Dad. My hatred for him grew. Mother sat in the kitchen, wilting like a dying flower. I thought that Dad was a wicked man to treat her like this. I never wanted to see him again. I decided that if I bumped into him on the street I would cross the road. If he spoke to me, I would ignore him.

On Sunday evening I went up the road to visit Nessan. I stayed in his house listening to Beatles records and discussing a job on the fishing boats until it was dark.

When I got home the first thing I noticed was a bouquet of beautiful flowers on the hall table. Dad was in the study, sitting in his black leather chair. My brother and sister were with him. They were laughing.

Mother waltzed past me from the kitchen carrying a tray with Dad's dinner on it. She didn't acknowledge me standing in the hallway with my outraged face. She looked happy.

I was no longer Man of the House. I had been dethroned by my own father. I was deeply confused. I didn't understand how things could have been sorted out so quickly. One day Dad had left for good. The next he was back in the black leather chair in the study as though nothing had happened.

The next morning at breakfast I wouldn't talk to Dad. Instead, I just glared at him. 'What's the matter with him?' Dad asked Mother.

Mother shrugged, 'Oh, don't mind him. You know what he's like.'

★

Dad could kick a football so hard it went through the hedge onto the road. There were holes all over the shrubbery from his shots at goal.

We sometimes played on the same side for two or three-a-sides against local kids. Dad stayed in goals and took fierce, unstoppable shots. I ran myself silly. It was a good combination and we always won.

Most of the time it was just me versus Dad. Our games always began with me kicking a ball about in the garden. Then Dad would appear in the front doorway. He'd watch for a while and then rapidly piston-walk down the steps to the front garden. He rarely said anything much, not even well done or good shot. The most he said was 'Oh' and that was only if he accidentally kicked a ball through the hedge onto the road. This would mean that I would have to run after it. Once I chased a ball halfway down Thormanby Road, and by the time I had returned with the ball, winded and sweaty, Dad had gone inside.

Dad loved soccer. He told me that he had once been a very fine goalkeeper. If he had practised a bit more, he could have played for his hometown team, Dundalk. The Christian Brothers in Dad's school used to punish kids who attended the Sunday soccer games in Oriel Park. They reckoned that attending soccer games was unpatriotic. Every Monday they would ask those boys who had been at the game on the previous day to put up their hands. To get boys to see the errors of their ways, the Brothers slapped those who had attended the match across the hands with a leather strap. This practice apparently ceased after my Dad's father marched into the school to confront the Brothers.

Dad brought me to Dalymount Park to see my first soccer game – Ireland versus Scotland in a friendly under sizzling floodlights. It was the first time I had been out with my dad at night (apart from adjudicating or first nights at the Abbey). The two of us rose to our feet, yelling our heads off when Don Givens scored for Ireland on his home debut. Colin Stein equalised for Scotland late in the same match. Dad didn't mind too much, he said it was a good goal and Scotland deserved it.

He took me to several matches after that, but that is the only one I remember.

One day when I was about fifteen I was kicking a ball about in the front garden with Nessan when Dad drove his Austin Cambridge through the wooden gates at the bottom of our driveway. We heard an enormous crunch and watched as slivers of white-painted wood rose into the air. We watched the Austin Cambridge roar up the drive and park. Dad got out and piston-walked up the path and then up the steps to the front door. Before going in he paused and looked at us as we stood gobsmacked in the garden. 'I was sick and tired of having to stop to open the shaggin' gates,' he said, and went in.

Later he made me clean up the broken wood. The white-painted gate stumps remained at the bottom of our driveway for the rest of our years in Howth.

★

My last soccer game with Dad was shortly after I began college. By then I was wearing flares all the time, the wider the better, and I'd grown my hair really long. It was difficult to play football when you were tramping about in trousers that felt like you were wearing parachutes on your ankles. Two local guys challenged us. 'We'll hockey you,' I told them.

They beat us easily. Dad wouldn't run or try to save shots. He remained rooted in goal and watched as the ball flew past. Occasionally, Dad whacked a shot over the hedge. I ran about but was easily outmanoeuvred by our opponents.

I was mad at Dad for letting me down. I didn't realise that Dad was too old now to dash about the way he used to when he played with me. He knew enough to stay put and not banjax himself for a meaningless game.

It hurt me that we had lost so badly, but it didn't bother Dad – or if it did, he didn't show it.

Afterwards, Dad piston-walked off up the steps to the house. I sat on the ball wondering what had gone wrong. I had had such faith in the dad–son combination and now it was gone. I realised that Dad was getting old and I was changing. The games in the front garden were over.

7

Rebel Without a Brain

For the first three years of secondary school, my class had mainly lay teachers. There was very little brutality. We were all relieved that we had avoided the fiercest and most feared Christian Brother, a crew-cut gorilla nicknamed Nelly who taught maths and Latin.

All the teachers had nicknames – Mao (because he looked Chinese and we reckoned that if the Chinese ever invaded Ireland they would pass over him as one of their own), Sparrow (because he looked like one), Buddha (because he looked like one), Boots (nobody could remember how he had come about his nickname, a source of great concern to Boots himself who was extremely curious), Piggy (because he looked like one) and Babs (the origins were uncertain, but the teacher was tall and skinny with a strong Dublin accent and it just seemed to fit).

At one stage we got a new temporary teacher who was fresh

out of teacher training college. He was accident prone and he quickly earned the nickname Praiseach (Irish for 'disaster'). Praiseach meant well but easily became exasperated and angry. Once he threw a duster at a boy only to hit the wrong lad, who immediately performed a big dramatic collapse to the floor, pretending to have been knocked unconscious. Another thrown duster rebounded off a boy's head and broke a window. Praiseach couldn't even get it together to walk around the classroom. He tripped over chairs, table legs and the corners of desks. His earnest efforts to control a class resulted in everyone either ignoring him or laughing at him. In a final desperate effort to get us to listen to him, he spoke to us in English about the joys of jazz music and of a trumpet player named Miles Davis. Mention of a trumpet inspired several boys to improvise trumpet solos by making loud squeaking noises. One boy placed his hand under an armpit and squeezed out trapped air in loud rhythmic parps that sounded like an outbreak of farting. 'It's the drums, sir,' he explained when Praiseach objected. Praiseach left at the end of that school year.

Our Latin teacher was nicknamed Flats. He was very old and had false teeth and sported an unconvincing wig that had once been blond, or at least fair, but now was a nuclear shade of orange. Sometimes he fell asleep in class and his wig began to slip. He woke up only when the wig tipped over his nose. Occasionally, a boy snuck up behind the dozing Flats to give the wig a helpful nudge.

After the moon landings, Seán, our handsome and unconventional teacher for Irish and civics, informed us that the whole Apollo 11 thing had been a fake. A friend of his brother worked in Hollywood and had worked on the very sound stage where the landings had been filmed. It was all a big scam to make the American public feel better and to enable US politicians to win elections. There was a lively debate, but Seán stuck to his story. Look at a James Bond movie, he told us. Sure you'd see the same kind of special effects.

That evening we went home to our parents to announce that the moon landings had been shot in a Hollywood studio. We knew because our teacher had told us so.

Within days a delegation of parents arrived in to meet Seán – but Seán stuck to his story. For some reason the parents found him charming and reasonable and there was no negative fallout. After the meeting Mother told me that Seán was probably right. She said that the Hollywood studios had the technology to make us believe anything. She said that Seán had eyes 'like green flex'.

For English we had Essential Joe, a tall man with a soft voice and a passion for words. Essential Joe was so named after his habit of saying 'essentially' before every second sentence. One day Joe set us an essay. The topic was the future. He said that if we wished, we could ignore the essay and write a short story instead as long as it was on the same subject. At that time I was still churning out the occasional red cashbook. I was also obsessed with the writings of Ray Bradbury, particularly his novels *Fahrenheit 451*, *Something Wicked This Way Comes* and *The Illustrated Man*, along with all of his science fiction short stories. Instead of an essay, I wrote a short story about four astronauts falling through space following the break-up of their spaceship. Bradbury had written a story on the same theme called 'Kaleidoscope', which was one of my favourites. I continued the storyline from the point where Bradbury had stopped, chronicling what happened to the four men as they descended into oblivion or entered a planet's atmosphere or were hit by space debris or whatever. Essential Joe loved my story and he read it out to the class. He told me that it was one of the best essays or stories that he had ever read. He encouraged me to continue to write. He told me that I had a terrific imagination. He said I was a natural writer.

I sat at my desk transfixed and astonished. I could feel a glow inside of me. I had never experienced praise like this before. I felt like a real writer now. The next day I dumped all my red cashbooks and started writing stories in big A4-sized manila copybooks. I wrote another story based upon the work of a writer I admired, Ambrose Bierce. I reinterpreted Bierce's *An Occurrence at Owl Creek Bridge*. I don't remember what I wrote but Essential Joe was impressed.

Essential Joe left Coláiste Mhuire after that year, but his encouragement had had a huge impact on me.

I kept the science fiction story until my late teens. Once I had started in UCD I threw my story into the bin, along with the Ambrose Bierce remix and all the red cashbooks I could find. I considered them juvenile. (Unbeknownst to me, my parents saved and hid a batch of my red cashbooks, including 'Satan's Saint' (parts one and two), which they presented to me on my fortieth birthday, along with my old teddy bear, Jojo.)

I still encountered difficulty learning, especially with maths and with algebra in particular. Throughout secondary school, whenever a teacher became sarcastic about my mathematical ability or criticised my grasp of algebra, my defence was to simply shut down. If they couldn't find a way to teach me, then I wouldn't make the effort to learn.

They thought I was thick, so I acted thick. I deliberately avoided studying maths or indeed any other subject that proved difficult to master. The only subject where I felt truly comfortable was English, mainly because of my love of reading but also because of Essential Joe's encouragement. I enjoyed history but I couldn't connect with the teaching, and again I had trouble with the Irish language.

Irish removed history from the real world and placed it inside some peculiar alternative Gaelic-language universe where everyone spoke Irish and only those events that directly affected Ireland or took place on Irish soil were truly worthy of consideration. The major events in world history seemed to revolve around an endless series of doomed uprisings by heroic Irish revolutionaries that were always ruthlessly suppressed by the English. The main historical effect of the Spanish Armada was that several Spanish galleons had wrecked themselves on Irish shores. The First World War was essentially a minor footnote to the 1916 Rising. Pádraig Pearse was a more important and influential world leader than Gandhi or Churchill. The only other world leader who was discussed in the same breath as the 1916 martyrs was John F Kennedy, and that was because his people came from Wexford and because he had visited Ireland in 1963. Whenever JFK was mentioned, it was always with a dark hint that a 'Sassenach' had been behind his assassination.

I developed and cultivated an unreasonable hatred of the Irish language and all things Gaelic. I refused to play Gaelic football or hurling. I occasionally played handball but if I noticed a Brother watching me I deliberately lost in case I got picked for the school team.

I began to turn myself into a rebel. I started hanging around with other boys I considered to be rebellious types, including a skinny boy with a high forehead nicknamed Marvo (his name in Irish was virtually unpronounceable and there was no point asking for his name in English because it couldn't be used in school) and another lad named Willie who hated Coláiste and all the teachers. Marvo and I and a bunch of other boys began to sneak out of school through the bicycle shed at lunchtimes. It was a quick dash from the bicycle shed entrance to the corner of the school and past into Granby Row and freedom. Rambling through the city at lunch break made me feel like a big boy. I was out in the big world where I didn't have to listen to or speak Irish. We just had to keep a lookout for wandering teachers and Christian Brothers.

In the week coming up to Hallowe'en we went to Moore Street Market in search of bangers, which were illegal. 'Want bangers, son?' an old lady on a fruit stall said quietly as we approached. We handed over our pooled lunch money and the old lady reached in her apron and came up with half a dozen bangers.

We let them off around town. We pushed a fizzing banger through a letterbox. We tossed another into a doorway. We were halfway down the next street by the time we heard the boom. We reserved the rest of the bangers for a china showroom on Abbey Street. Three of four bangers tossed in at the same time produced a series of glorious booms followed by rattling china. Disappointingly, there were no big smashes. We were also disappointed that we weren't chased.

A boy named Barry came with us on some of our voyages into the city. He nicknamed himself Barrance and delighted in a new kind of language which was derived from existing Dublin slang as well as from the pop radio and magazines. Anything Barrance liked was 'fab' or 'the gear'. Other stuff that pleased him was termed 'rapid'. People didn't live in houses, they lived in 'gaffs'. Boys never got into fights, instead they had 'claims' – if they lost the fight they got 'claimed'. Anything he didn't like was 'brutal'. An amount of money over a pound was labelled 'fifty million quid' as in, 'I couldn't afford to buy a Beatles LP, it was fifty million quid.'

Barrance sprayed out his colourful expressions in a cheerful Dublin accent. I was so impressed that I went to great pains to develop a Dublin accent like Barrance's, a task in which I was reasonably successful. People who heard me speaking with my school friends often mistook me for a kid from the inner city. Barrance had a special swagger that coupled with his cheeky grin made him the outstanding personality in our group. He also seemed to be born lucky. He was never caught for any mischief he was involved in and he was never blamed for any wrongdoing. His luck and nonchalance gained him enormous respect as well as a great reputation. I thought he was the funniest, most original and impressive fellow I had ever met.

On one of our excursions we discovered a playground near a block of flats that was always deserted at lunchtime. The playground had the usual kid stuff – swings and roundabouts and the like – but it also had a seesaw that we used to play a rough and dangerous game called bronco riding. Bronco riding was very simple. A boy sat on one end of the seesaw while the rest of us tried our best to knock him off by slamming the other end of the seesaw into the concrete as hard and as fast as possible. Nobody lasted longer than five slams. Most fell off after two.

Best of all, adjoining the playground there was a full-sized concrete soccer pitch with iron goals. We picked teams and played tournaments. I kept the results and goal scorers in one of my red cashbooks. One day a laconic, easy-going chap named Boyle wandered over to casually enquire how many goals he had scored in the ten or eleven games he had played in. I told him he'd scored once, while Dignam, Boyle's mortal enemy, had scored seven. He was outraged and in the next game played like a maniac to score five goals. He ended up as the leading goal scorer in our mini league.

To make the journey to the playground more interesting, we climbed onto a high wall that stretched from the street across the road from the back of our school to the CIÉ bus depot about a mile away. We walked along the wall's narrow top, where keeping your balance was tricky. On one side of the wall lay a footpath where people occasionally looked up at us. On the other side were people's houses and back gardens. We took great delight in staring at people as they cooked their lunches or busied themselves in studies or back bedrooms.

People yelled at us. Irate homeowners greatly resented glancing through their back windows to find themselves under scrutiny by a group of smug boys. Several came outside to get us to climb down from the wall, but we always scarpered and were usually well past by the time they emerged from their kitchens or back bedrooms. Once we spied a couple kissing in their bedroom. We wailed and hooted until they looked up and saw us and then we waved. Later, we told everyone back in school that we had seen a couple having sex. Next lunchtime, our little group of adventurous walkers had doubled. Sadly, this time the couple had drawn the bedroom curtains.

There was something tremendously rewarding about being able to walk along a dangerous narrow ledge and piss off adults at the same time. I loved being a daredevil. I liked anything that was different and a bit dangerous. It was a miracle that none of us ever fell off the wall or got hurt bronco riding or messing about in the playground. Somehow, none of us ever got caught sneaking either in or out of the bicycle shed.

Sometimes for a change at lunch breaks, Marvo and I and a few others climbed onto the roof of the science building at the back of the school to explore the rooftops of Parnell Square. We found a skylight on the roof of the Hugh Lane Gallery that was never locked or else the lock was broken. We climbed down into a dark storeroom. Then we snuck into the top floors of the gallery itself. The gallery offered free admission, but that wasn't the point. It was far more thrilling to enter and exit the building through the roof skylight than to walk in the front door. Marvo maintained that sneaking in gave us a better appreciation of the art exhibits, particularly the ones kept in the storeroom, which for some reason were mostly nude paintings of women. We often brought flashlights and snuck into the storeroom to eat our sandwiches, shining the flashlights at paintings as we discussed the artists' representations of women's nude bodies. The nude paintings were too old fashioned and, to our eyes, too unrealistic to be really sexy, but we all agreed that they were better to look at than some of the modern works to be found in the main gallery. We despised one main gallery exhibit in particular, a huge canvas featuring a big glob of orange paint that reminded us of a toddler's attempt at painting the sun.

Then one day Marvo announced that he was leaving. He promised to write, but I didn't believe him. Now another friend was about to disappear. At least this time I had had some warning.

Barrance also left, along with his friend Burkie and several other boys I really liked. I palled around with Willie, a dark, good-looking kid who was a swimming champion. Willie said he was going to leave as well. He was going to head for Morocco to smoke dope and sleep with women. I decided that I would go with him. For weeks, we made plans. If we sold all our albums, we'd have enough money to get to London. Then we'd work there for a while to earn enough money for plane tickets. We would make it to Morocco before the summer. Neither of us saw any point sitting our Inter Cert exams.

First, though, we had to leave school. We decided that the best plan was to get ourselves expelled. That way there would be no going back.

Willie came out to Howth and met some of my friends. A boy named Smedley said that he would come into town and help us get expelled, even though he was working and didn't go to school, or so he said anyway.

As we explored various plots, I felt as though I was starring in my own action movie. I had become a hero from one of the stories that used to get passed around in the days of the Authors' Club. I had no idea what I was going to do in Morocco. I had never smoked dope and I was sure that Willie hadn't either, but then again Willie had done a lot more things than me so I couldn't be sure. The only thing I knew for sure was that I hated school and despised the Irish language and I needed to change my life. I was a rebel and this was a chance to prove it. Morocco seemed like a good way to do that, though deep down I began to suspect that the whole plan was probably just talk. It was bound to fizzle out.

Willie didn't turn up for school for a few days. I figured that the plan was off. Then one morning I found him waiting for me outside the Candy Shop around the corner from school. The plan was still on. Suddenly I was terrified. Now I was on the spot.

I wanted to say that I had had second thoughts, but I couldn't speak. We made plans to get expelled the next morning. I was to contact Smedley and bring him along. Willie seemed full of bravado. I probably appeared confident to Willie, but I was putting on a big front. I was totally lost. I didn't want to be a rebel any more. I had no notion of what I was doing or why I really wanted to quit school and go to Morocco, a country I knew nothing about except that it was very hot all the time and that hippies went there. I had become caught up in a silly scheme that was now about to change into a reality I could not handle. I did not have the courage to call the whole thing off or to walk away from it.

Somehow I got through the day in school. That night I got in touch with Smedley and the big plan was set. I don't remember much about the rest of the night or the next morning.

Willie, Smedley and me met outside the main entrance to Coláiste Mhuire at nine the next morning. We smirked at all the other poor boys that were not going to Morocco with us. We refused to go to class and wandered through the empty yard and then traipsed along the deserted corridors. We could hear the noise of classes being conducted and the normal activities of school. We lasted until the eleven o'clock break. At the sound of the bell, we suddenly began to run madly around the school yelling, for some reason, the word 'potatoes'. We ended up in the school hall, where we made a mad dash for the stairs to the main entrance. On the top of the stairs we took it in turns to leap over a cleaning lady who was on her hands and knees washing the wooden floor. Then we ran down the stairs through the thronging students and out the main doors of the school to the outside and down the street.

We hung around town for the rest of the morning, intoxicated by our daring and rebelliousness. We ended up in Stephen's Green looking out across the lake at the ducks.

Gradually, the feeling of euphoria wore off.

Smedley went off to work and Willie went to meet someone. I walked down to Abbey Street and caught the thirty-one bus home. On the way to Howth, the reality of what I had done troubled me. I began to feel guilty as well as incredibly stupid. By the time I got home I knew that I wasn't a hero in some made-up tale. I had made a huge mistake and turned my life into a complete disaster. I didn't want to go to Morocco any more. I wanted to go back to school and say sorry to the cleaning lady.

That evening I confessed everything to my mother. I began by saying that there had been a bit of trouble in school. I then told her that the school didn't want me anymore. She got on the phone to the school and I was sent to my room. I was banned from ever having any contact with either Smedley or Willie again.

Next week I went back to Coláiste Mhuire. I got a brief lecture from a Christian Brother. Later I apologised to the cleaning lady for jumping over her.

I went back to my class and it was as though the big day of rebellion had never happened. Nobody said anything to me. Hardly anybody had noticed our weird behaviour.

Willie never returned to school. I didn't see him for many years. In the late seventies we bumped into each other in Freebird Records on Grafton Street. We were adults now and had little to say to one another. I didn't have the nerve to ask if he had ever made it to Morocco.

I got involved in a lot of mischief in school. I enjoyed the messing, but I also saw it as a way of fighting back against the Brothers. The day-of-rebellion incident was a lucky escape, one I probably didn't deserve. I made a vow to keep out of trouble in the future.

It didn't last long.

I hated Coláiste Mhuire and the institutionalised viciousness of some of the Christian Brothers. On most mornings throughout primary school and for the first three or four years of secondary, I arrived in school fearful and lacking in confidence. I had bad nightmares. I often faked illness to get out of going to school. Sometimes it worked and I got to stay home to make a miraculous recovery by the time *Jackanory* came on TV. Sometimes I was sent to school even when I really was sick.

I felt trapped in the world of the Brothers, where even Gaelic was used as a weapon. Not being from the country and not being fluent in Irish were held up as deficiencies of character that the Brothers were trying their best to correct. And if that meant occasionally resorting to physical punishment to beat the alien attitudes and language out of a boy, then so be it – it could only make for a better boy. The Brothers appeared to want to churn out boys who would become useful participants in a new Irish society that would be entirely Gaelic speaking. An underlying message was that this new nation would develop a fine, upstanding army of ex-Coláiste Mhuire handball champions who would march up North and kick the Brits into the sea.

In school I found it easy to be creative and enthusiastic when it came to playing pranks. I had great confidence in my powers of mischief and almost none in my ability to learn from the curriculum that the school taught.

★

In the Inter Cert I somehow achieved four honours and two passes. Not brilliant, but slightly better than the average. I failed maths which had come as no surprise to anyone.

I took whatever punishment was meted out, usually a few belts across the hands with a leather strap. I affected a nonchalant attitude, cracking jokes afterwards and refusing to take things seriously. The truth was that I expected one day to be badly beaten by one of the more violent Brothers.

The strange thing was that while I dreaded the lashes across the palms with a leather strap or occasional twisted ears or slaps across the back of the legs with a ruler, it was the psychological taunting that affected me most. The Brothers liked to make a show of a boy in front of his friends. They liked to make a boy feel bad about himself.

Once, Nelly, a gorilla with a buzz cut who taught maths and biology, dressed me down for getting my sums wrong.

'You're a long, lanky, lazy *liúdramán*,' he said in English.

Everyone laughed.

'What are ye?'

'I'm a long, lanky, lazy *liúdramán*,' I repeated.

More nervous laughs, even from my pals.

He then said it in Gaelic and made me repeat that.

He smiled. 'Now ye know what ye are in two tongues,' Nelly said.

Nelly called me names anytime he felt like it for the final years of secondary school.

At first I shrugged it off, but eventually it got to me. I tried to make sure that I never made eye contact with Nelly.

Long. Lanky. Lazy. *Liúdramán*.

I felt ashamed of my height. I really did feel that I was lazy – it explained why I was useless at maths. I had no idea what a *liúdramán* was. I knew that it must be really savage because it was a word that Nelly had reserved exclusively for me.

Being tall was now a liability instead of a defence. I was six foot two in Third Year. Whenever mischief kicked off, I was the first one the teachers saw when they spun around from the blackboard. I practised hunching down in my seat, but that only got me sent to the line for slouching. I often got blamed when someone else broke wind spectacularly or fired a piece of chalk at the plastic chandelier to make a soft yet satisfying ding and thus confuse the teacher.

One of the most fiendish bits of mischief involved cautiously striking a match under the desk to set fire to the end of a chopped up piece of shoelace. The smouldering shoelace was then carefully placed on the shoulder of an unsuspecting class-mate to slowly but relentlessly burn through jumper fabric onto bare flesh, eventually provoking a surprised yell from the victim along with momentary mayhem in the class. I don't know who thought that one up, but it ruined a lot of jumpers.

I saw mischief as a method of livening up a drab and dreary school regime, as well as a tactic in my fight against the Brothers. I accepted the occasional miscarriage of justice as part of the price you had to pay.

We had Barreller for geography. He was a hefty, apparently jolly Christian Brother with an enduring grin. He looked a lot like Herman Goering. He had a strange way of pronouncing words that began with *s* coupled with an inability to say diffi-cult place names such as Saskatchewan, which in his mouth came out as 'Siskat-kat-kat-chewy' if it came out at all. He also mixed English phrases with Irish, giving his speeches a strange, almost surreal quality, like a type of pidgin Gaelic. '*Duirt mé libh* that I want *cuinneas*' ('I told you I wanted quiet') was a favourite phrase. 'I said I want *dairíre* (sincerity)' was another of his most celebrated comments, and much imitated by the class mimics.

Barreller had a likeable side and would have been a memo-rable – even a good – teacher if it hadn't been for his violent tendencies as well as his fondness for feeling up young boys.

Barreller liked to take boys up to his desk and put his hand in their pockets, a practice known as Barreller's pocket bil-liards. Sometimes he openly fondled boys' necks and backs and occasionally their bums, chortling at the same time as though thrusting his hand deep into a boy's pocket or up under his shirt was just harmless fun. He liked to sit boys on his knee and jockey them about as though showing them how to ride a horse. One boy returned to his desk after such an ordeal. 'He had a horn on him,' the boy told me. 'I could feel it sticking into me through his trousers.'

He only tried it with me once. He brought me up to stand alongside him where he sat behind his work table. He spouted some rubbish about tall fellows having longer backbones and more peculiar bone structures, and that gave him an excuse to lift my shirt and put his hand up. At first he confined his hands to exploring my back and I went numb trying to imagine that I was somewhere else while at the same time hoping that he wasn't going to touch my bum or my groin. I felt humiliated in front of my classmates. I had watched some of them endure the same treatment – now it was my turn.

When Barreller suddenly dropped his hand I pulled away. He just laughed, as though it was the exact reaction he had been seeking. He didn't try to stop me. He told me to sit down. I was probably too tall for him to bother with. He liked smaller lads.

Barreller once stopped me on the stairs for a quiet word. He asked me if I had ever seen a certain boy's 'yoke', as he put it. I told him that I had not. 'Not even during gym class in the changing rooms?' he asked. 'No,' I said. He named other boys, asking me if I had seen their 'yokes' when we were all lined up at the urinals. Again, I said that I had not. He looked worried for a moment, as though he had been expecting a different answer, and then he dismissed me.

There were stories about Barreller luring boys down to the bicycle shed at the break or after school, where he supposedly 'queered' them. Several times I heard him invite boys to stay behind after school to visit him in his rooms, where he offered to show them his special atlas. If anyone accepted his invitation, I never heard about it.

Barreller kept a large leather in his back pocket. He whacked me several times for talking in class or not doing homework. One beating left my hands sore for days. A boy told me that the trick was to excuse yourself just before the punishment, go to the toilets and wee all over your hands. Then when you got hit it didn't hurt as much. Other boys claimed to have managed the feat, but I could never pluck up the courage. The thought of pissing on my hands was almost as unappealing as the beating itself.

Barreller was depraved, but there was a cartoon quality to him because of his mangled language and his odd mannerisms – except maybe to those boys he abused.

★

There was nothing cartoonish or likeable about Nelly. Nelly used a bamboo cane as well as a leather, and always made sure to aim it for the joints and knuckles so that it would really sting. I once saw Nelly inflict savage punishment on a boy who kept moving his hand at the last second, causing the bamboo to glance off. To get the boy to keep his hands steady, Nelly slapped him across the face. Nelly then resumed his bamboo beating. He stopped only when the boy was bent over and howling.

At one stage, possibly at the end of Third Year or perhaps at the beginning of Fifth, Nelly decided to teach us the facts of life during the weekly biology lesson. He unfolded a chart of the human body – a medicinal and rather bloody-looking caricature that depicted a person's entrails and other inner workings in vivid colour. Nelly then held up a small toy bicycle. He told us, in Gaelic, that he was going to talk to us about *gnéas* (sex) and that if anyone sniggered or made silly noises he would beat them to a lump of raw meat.

He explained that whenever a boy rode a bicycle the lower part of his body became stimulated. With a bamboo cane Nelly indicated the human groin on the body chart. He said that the male member can become aroused when stimulated. When that happened it grew stiff. When it got stiff, it stood up. If some fluid should issue from the tip of this erect part of the body when a boy was riding downhill on a bicycle, then that was perfectly natural and nothing to be ashamed of. Abruptly, Nelly's face darkened and he slapped the chart a swift clatter with his bamboo. But if a boy put his hand down there and helped that fluid to issue forth, then that was a mortal sin.

Nobody cracked a smile. Nelly stared at us for a long while to check if anyone would weaken.

Somehow we all remained stone faced, even though we had just been informed by a supposedly reliable source that sex only happened to a guy when he became excited while speeding downhill on a bicycle and usually when he was alone.

After a few moments of glaring at us, Nelly folded up the chart and gave us something else to do.

We didn't know much about sex, but now we knew even less.

One day during maths Nelly picked on Tony, a tall, bright, solid guy who was a good student and naturally quiet in class. Tony refused to back down. Nelly told Tony to get up. Tony stood up. Nelly slapped Tony hard across the face with his open palm. The smack could be heard in the classes below. Nelly stared at Tony. Tony stared back and told him not to do that again. Nelly slapped him again, harder this time. The confrontation between a large Christian Brother dressed in black and a sixteen-year-old boy seemed perverse. I genuinely believed that Nelly was about to hurt Tony so badly that he would be hospitalised. I had never seen anyone get hit that hard by an adult. Not even in movies. Nelly hit Tony again and Tony's head rocked back.

Somehow Tony remained standing. In soft words, Tony told Nelly that he would not dare hit him outside school. Nelly glared at Tony. It seemed that he was daring Tony to hit him back so he could have an excuse to expel him. Nelly said that he would meet Tony after school to settle this anytime and anyplace that Tony wanted. Before Tony could reply Nelly struck him again. This one sounded like a gunshot. Tony remained standing.

Then Nelly walked back to the blackboard and continued the lesson as though nothing had happened.

After the class Tony's cheeks were red and bruised looking, but he remained defiant. He had faced Nelly and retained his dignity and composure. He had won a small but crucial victory under extreme provocation. I doubted if I would have been as brave.

★

The Head Brother, O'Cathnithe (or Canny), took us for Latin and religion. He was a diminutive, belligerent gargoyle who could be charming but had no compunction about punching a boy or slashing someone across the face with a leather strap. He administered several beatings. He whacked my hands and legs. He slapped other boys and brought tears to their eyes, but nobody cried. Not breaking down was considered the only way to fight back. Never let the bastards see you crack.

Canny once raised his fist to my face and hissed, '*Cuirfidh mé mo dhorn siar in do bhéal, a bhuco.*' ('I'll ram my fist down your throat, my boyo.') My offence was to have scrawled Crystal Palace, the name of my favourite team, on the cover of my religion reader.

One afternoon during civics, Canny led a discussion on the meanings behind Gaelic surnames. Beaming, he boasted that the literal translation of his own name, O'Cathnithe, was 'battle champion'. In his own mind, his dealings with us were battles and he won them all.

He made Barreller look compassionate.

I heard the sarcastic voices of Barreller, Nelly and Canny whenever I did my homework or studied or read a book. I felt that I could do nothing right. I felt that I could not learn. After a while, this attitude hardened into a refusal to learn maths or anything else.

In maths class I often tuned out altogether. While everyone else was absorbing algebra, I made lists in my copybook of my favourite rock and rollers – Ten Years After, The Allman Brothers Band, Atomic Rooster, Colosseum, Thin Lizzy, Rory Gallagher, Frank Zappa, The Doors, The Groundhogs, If, Gentle Giant, Procul Harum, Gnidrolog (I have never met anyone else who liked or who has even heard of Gnidrolog), Joni Mitchell, Renaissance... Making lists of my favourite artists made me feel better and more in control of my situation, if only temporarily or until I got caught. I could recall the line-ups of every band I liked. I couldn't work out the simplest equation in algebra, but I could tell you who had been the original bassist in Deep Purple (Nic Simper). I could recite the line-up of the Crystal Palace team (John Jackson in goals to Gerry Queen and Alan Birchenal up front), and indeed any football team in the English First Division, but once it came to maths and long division, I was lost. When I wasn't making lists, I daydreamed about playing lead guitar in a rock band.

Once, when Barreller discovered a list of my favourite writers on the back of my geography copybook, he made me read it out to the class. 'Ian Fleming, John Creasey, Denis Wheatley, Herman Hesse, Jean Bruce, Dylan Thomas, Ray Bradbury...'

As penance he instructed me to find out where these writers lived and give an account of the agricultural situation in their areas. It was an inspired idea, but I deliberately refused to carry it out. I wanted to be taught by a teacher who was not a violent pervert. After a while, Barreller either forgot that he had asked me or decided against following through.

In refusing to learn I thought I was taking a stand against a repressive regime, but in truth all I was doing was undermining my own education. My stubbornness left huge gaps in my learning. I blamed myself for my attitude, but I seemed to have had a learning disability, particularly with regard to maths and Irish. I also struggled to make sense of French and Latin homework. I became exasperated by having to translate into English and then Irish and then back to French or Latin again. I tuned out of so many classes that my English was affected. I ended up with a freewheeling, somewhat improvisational approach to grammar and syntax.

The sarcastic voices followed me home at weekends. I heard them in my head, criticising my clothes and my long hair and my passion for rock music and soccer and strange writers. I found it hard to accept that criticism of any kind was anything other than a personal attack. This feeling persisted for years after I left Coláiste.

On the day that I received my honours degree in English and History from UCD, I stood outside with my parents while somebody snapped a photo. I couldn't relax to enjoy the moment because I expected a Christian Brother's hand to land suddenly upon my shoulder while a gruff voice downgraded my achievement. I would not have been surprised if my degree had been plucked from my hands because the university had received reports that I wasn't completely fluent in Gaelic or because I had failed maths in the Inter or that I had once jumped over a cleaning lady in the school canteen.

I saw all Christian Brothers, as well as some teachers, as enemies. I don't recall any parent complaining about the way their kids were treated. Nor did I know of any boy who had been withdrawn from school because of the brutality or the bad teaching. Whenever I raised the issue with my parents they dismissed my claims. The fact that I wasn't beaten very often or that most punishments tended to be half a dozen slaps across the hands with a leather or bamboo was accepted and regarded normal.

My years in Coláiste Mhuire convinced me that many of the adults who had power over me were violent, lazy or incompetent or all three together. Some were evil men who should not have been put in charge of children or teenagers. I developed a mistrust of authority and authority figures that lasted well into my thirties and still haunts me.

There were only two women teachers in secondary school. Monica was a straight-talking, no-nonsense type who taught maths. Lucy was a gentle, dreamy brunette who taught French. Quite a few of us developed a crush on Lucy, who was extremely petite as well as pretty. She sometimes wore miniskirts. One day a competition began amongst us to see who would be the first to deduce the colour of Lucy's knickers. Biros dropped to the floor, accompanied by copybooks and French readers. Schoolbags toppled over. Any excuse to bend down and get a good look was used. If Lucy noticed our shenanigans, she gracefully ignored them.

We tried the same tactics with Monica when she arrived in wearing a miniskirt. After the fifth or sixth dropped biro, she fixed us in a steely glare. 'For your information,' she announced calmly, 'they're red.'

★

When I was sixteen Dad brought me to America with him. He figured that I was running wild at home and was concerned that if he didn't take me with him I might not be at home when he got back.

The first thing I noticed after landing at the airport in New York was the astonishing heat. It seemed to go right into your lungs and made it hard to breathe.

The second thing I noticed was that a great many American girls were as tall as me. They were all blonde and tanned – proper, healthy-looking, nut-brown skin tones with no bright-orange hues.

We stopped off for a night in New York and we saw *Jesus Christ Superstar* at the Mark Hellinger Theatre. The special effects were spectacular. The best bit was when Judas hanged himself by a noose that lifted him into the air past our seats in the balcony and higher to eventually disappear into the darkness below the theatre's high ceiling. At the interval we bumped into a girl from our neighbourhood. She came up to say hello and chat with us like we were on Howth Strand.

In the hotel the next morning Dad bought a newspaper from an old man at a concession stand in the lobby. The old man was Irish and he and Dad began a conversation in Gaelic. When he was finished one of the porters approached Dad to politely enquire what language Dad and the news vendor had been speaking. The porter and his friend had had a wager on it. Dad told him and the porter looked pleased – he had just won fifty bucks.

Later Dad had to meet someone, so he gave me some dollars and told me I could go for a ramble around Times Square. He told me to be careful.

Wandering around Times Square was the first time in my life that I felt like an adult. I was in New York wearing my best denims with dollars in my pocket. In Ireland everyone was white or ruddy coloured. Here I was surrounded by people of every shade. At first I found it a bit intimidating, but after a while I loved being in the middle of the New York mix. I felt that I had arrived into the real world. Every store seemed to be playing 'Lean on Me' by Bill Withers. I decided to go and see a new movie, *Shaft,* that was playing in a cinema on Times Square. I paid in and found my seat in the darkness. The first feature was rubbish. It was about some kid who was trying to save his father's corner shop in a small town in the mid-west. When it was over the house lights came up. I looked around. The cinema was almost full. All I could see were afro hairstyles. I was the only white face in the audience. Everyone else was either black or Hispanic and definitely male. I tried not to catch anyone's eye. I watched the movie with an uneasy feeling in my gut. I half expected to be knifed by some pimp. All the prejudices I thought I didn't have came through. It didn't help when the audience let out a huge roar of approval every time Shaft blew away some honky. I wanted Dad to come and take me home. I wished he hadn't let me go off on my own.

The reason we were in America was Dad's gig lecturing in Irish theatre at Carlton College, Minnesota. We lived in a fine house in Osceola Avenue in St Paul/Minneapolis. The house belonged to a nice couple named de Long. I hung around with their son, John, who had just returned from Vietnam, where he had been wounded. John was about twenty. He had stepped on a mine and been told that he would not walk again. That was a year ago. Now he was water-skiing barefoot. He had curly black hair and a thick moustache. He had a beautiful, tanned, Irish-American girlfriend named Jane but they had had a row and weren't speaking. John didn't take crap from anyone, but he looked out for me and brought me around with him.

John took me cruising one night. We slowed down to speak to a couple of hippy chicks who were walking home. John convinced the girls to come for a drive with us. 'What age is he?' a hippy chick said, indicating me.

'He's older than me,' John replied.

We went back to John's apartment. John brought a hippy chick with him into the bedroom. He wanted to show her his water pipe. I grappled with the other hippy chick on the sofa. I had no idea what I was doing and she quickly became irritated. We could hear the sounds of enjoyment emanating from the darkened bedroom.

'What if we turn the lights off?' I said to the hippy chick.

'What if we don't,' she answered.

Later John dropped the girls home. The grumpy hippy chick and I sat in the back and pretended to be fascinated by the scenery.

On the Fourth of July we were invited to go on a boat cruise around one of the lakes. Dad and the right-wing lawyer who owned the boat got into an argument about Vietnam. The lawyer felt that the US needed to win the war quickly with maximum force; Dad argued that the US had no business being in Vietnam. They ended up shaking hands. Later the lawyer approached me where I sat drinking beer in the shade of the cabin.

'Your Dad's a good guy,' the lawyer said. 'We don't agree on things but we can talk about it, and that's what this country is all about.' Then he gave me a grass joint rolled in what looked like a five-dollar bill. I was reluctant to smoke it until he showed me a packet of specially made imitation dollar bill cigarette papers.

Dad's students adored him, especially the girls – I was too young for them to be bothered with. I asked Dad if he was tempted by all the tanned, blonde beauties. He didn't seem surprised by my question. 'No, son. Your mother's enough for me.'

8

Sex, Drugs and Ceilí Music

I tried to hold on to a basketball while being dangled headfirst halfway out of a third-storey window by my classmates. Below, rows of parked cars were lined up like an honour guard waiting for me to fall. I could see traffic chugging past on busy Parnell Square.

Then my classmates started tickling me.

We had been messing with a basketball in our Fifth Year classroom during morning break. (For some reason, basketball had qualified as an 'Irish' sport in Coláiste Mhuire.) Three or four boys grabbed me and pushed me to the window. They thought it was great gas to hold me halfway out with my feet off the floor. The only way to escape the tickling and avoid falling out the window was to get rid of the basketball.

So I let go.

I watched the basketball plummet three stories to rebound majestically from the bonnet of Mr Judge's Rolls Royce. I saw the basketball bounce off down the street before it finally rolled around the corner, narrowly missing the front wheels of a bus. The bus braked with a screech.

We all dashed to our seats. The only thing to do now was to wait for the investigation.

Mr Judge taught English, but he was quite well known for writing Irish-language songs as entries to the *National Song Contest*. He nearly always won a money prize and at least one of his songs was picked to represent Ireland at the *Eurovision Song Contest*. Somewhere along the line, Mr Judge had got himself a Rolls that he always parked directly outside the main entrance to the school.

Now I had basketball-bombed his pride and joy.

For the rest of that morning, those of us who had been involved in the incident remained subdued and anxious. I was the most worried. If we were caught then I was the one who would really get in trouble because I had actually dropped the basketball. Denting the car of a teacher with the gym basketball at break time could get me expelled. I had lost an item of school property. I had also endangered the lives of the public.

The investigating team reached our class late that afternoon. The team consisted of an excitable Mr Judge accompanied by a menacingly silent Brother Piggy. When they asked if anyone knew about the basketball that had been thrown out of a school window, there was a long silence. Eventually, I raised my hand. Mr Judge beckoned me to accompany him outside.

Judge was a small, dapper man with receding hair. He sported thick-rimmed glasses with strong lenses. He had a reputation for being a stern but excellent teacher. We had only known him as an occasional replacement when other teachers were ill. On one such occasion he had arrived into the classroom unnoticed and observed our antics in silence for a few moments. Then he had suddenly yelled 'knickers'. The class hushed. Everyone looked at Judge, who immediately went to the blackboard and picked up a piece of chalk. 'Now that I've got your attention, we can begin,' he said.

Judge asked why I had decided to drop a basketball onto the bonnet of his car. I explained that I had been carrying a basketball in the classroom and that I had dropped it accidentally. As I went to pick it up, the ball had hit me on the knee and bounced out of the window before I could catch it.

When Mr Judge stopped laughing, he admonished me for behaving recklessly. Did I not realise that I could have caused an accident? He didn't say anything about damage to his car. He sent me back to class and told me not to do it again. I was grateful that he was so gracious. He could have had me suspended or expelled. For once, my misdemeanour did not get me brutalised by the Christian Brothers. I had been expecting at least a few whacks across the hands from a leather strap.

The next morning, boys from other classes pointed at me in the yard. 'There's Mac Anna. He bombed Judgie's Roller with a basketball.'

Afterwards I noticed that Judge parked his car further down the street, away from the top-floor windows.

★

There were just sixteen boys in our class throughout Fifth Year. We bonded easily. Nobody ever ratted on another boy, no matter how serious the mischief. The camaraderie was genuine and unusual. Arriving into class each morning, I felt as though I had fifteen close friends. The social aspect of school was an exciting and rewarding experience. It was the only compensation that I derived from my time in Coláiste Mhuire. From Fifth Year onwards, I sincerely looked forward to going to school each morning.

I spent most of my breaks discussing books and music with Tadhg, and sometimes Cian. Tadhg was the class guru and the other boys in the class were respectful of his knowledge and individual stance. He seemed to know a lot about spiritual matters, particularly Eastern philosophy and faith. He was quiet and thoughtful, but he loved mischief. He was determined to find an alternative way in the world rather than settle for the usual crap of a nine-to-five office job.

Tadhg was interested in astral travel. He told me that it was possible to leave one's body while sleeping to travel in the astral plane – a parallel spirit universe where a person could have many extraordinary experiences and learn how to develop a stronger spiritual persona. He lent me a book, *Astral Projection and Out of Body Experiences*, by some American doctor.

I was fascinated. I learned that every human being possessed a visible aura, a sort of surrounding overcoat of light complete with colour changes to reflect mood and character. By training yourself, it was possible to see a person's aura and interpret its colours. Tadhg and I spent lots of time practising 'seeing' one another's auras. A large amount of green in a person's aura was considered good. Too much red or orange meant that you were dealing with an angry or vicious person. We swore we could see each other's auras, and those of others in the class. We didn't bother looking for the auras of any of the teachers. We figured most of them were past redemption.

At home I nearly went cross-eyed staring at myself in the mirror, trying to figure out what colours shimmered gently around my naked body.

Now that I had convinced myself that I could see auras, I decided that I was ready for astral travel. I promised to visit Tadhg at night. He said he'd be looking out for me.

That night I lay in bed with my arms at my sides and tried to leave my body. I fell asleep and had vivid dreams about flying. The next morning in school, Tadhg admitted that he might have seen something in his room, but he couldn't be sure. For many nights we tried to visit each other in our respective homes, but nothing much came of it. To maintain our enthusiasm, we admitted to brief 'sightings' of 'something'. Astral projection wasn't dangerous, but there were demons and other horrors in the astral plane and it was best to go slowly and know what you were doing rather than plunge in. There was a miniscule risk that a rash or inexperienced astral traveller could tangle with a nasty entity in the spirit world and become possessed. But you would have to be really stupid or spectacularly unlucky to end up like the girl in *The Exorcist*.

Tadhg encouraged me to keep practising. Achieving entry to the spiritual plane wasn't something that you could expect right away. He told me stories about places that he had visited in his spirit body. There were times when he wasn't sure if he was actually in the astral plane or simply experiencing a particularly vivid dream. One trick was to become aware that you were dreaming without actually waking up. Once you had made yourself conscious within your own dream, it should be possible to control your actions and really begin to zoom about on the astral plane.

After several months' effort I had about as much success with astral projection as I did with maths, but at least my nightmares went away and I felt calmer in school.

Cian had long, blond hair and looked like an attractive girl. He wore sandals and hippy clothes. He reminded me of the boy from the poster of *Death in Venice*.

The first time I saw him in the yard I thought he was a girl. Now that I was in the same class and becoming friends with him I wasn't sure how I felt. For a time I even thought I fancied him. Maybe I was gay and didn't know it. I was a bit confused around Cian.

Most of us in the class claimed to have girlfriends but in reality few of us seemed to have had much experience with the opposite sex. We didn't know much about drugs, though some of us had puffed on joints at parties. I had tried dope and it had had no effect whatsoever. I preferred the tipped cigars that some of us bought in the Candy Shop after school and smoked on the way down O'Connell Street to make ourselves feel cool and adult. We swapped stories about how acid or LSD raised your consciousness or else made you laugh uncontrollably for twenty-four hours. We were intrigued, but we were on safer ground discussing the beneficial qualities of a pint of Guinness.

Cian, though, seemed somewhat removed from such concerns. He had an air about him of being above worldly matters. He appeared more self-contained and secure than the rest of us. He seemed to need less from the world than we did. He told us once that he wanted to become a monk, preferably in a silent order.

Tadhg, Cian and I hung around together and talked about astral travel. We read and exchanged unusual and interesting books, such as *The Glass Bead Game* and *Siddhartha* by Herman Hesse and *A Confederate General at Big Sur* by Richard Brautigan. *Zen and the Art of Motorcycle Maintenance* by Robert Pirsig was another favourite.

I pretended to like Hesse, but in reality I found the writing boring and occasionally, as in *The Glass Bead Game*, insufferable. But I liked *Siddhartha* because I was captivated by its depiction of a young man on a spiritual quest. I thought *Steppenwolf* was cool, not just because it was an intriguing and unusual tale but also because it had inspired the name of the rock band who sang 'Born to be Wild'.

We hung around the Candy Shop at lunchtimes, hoping to run into girls from Scoil Caitríona. We got friendly with some. I was always too shy to ask a girl out. I was OK once a conversation started, but I was useless at initiating contact. Tadhg was more confident, and girls seemed to like him. Girls didn't know what to make of Cian. Some probably thought he was one of them in disguise.

★

One St Patrick's night Tadhg and I and about a dozen others attempted to gatecrash a special party for a bunch of American cheerleaders at the Gresham Hotel. Word had it that American cheerleaders were easy to seduce, especially on St Patrick's Day.

We failed to get past the bouncers. Even a plea that we were a special goodwill delegation from the only Irish-language boys' school in Dublin cut no ice.

Somehow we ended up hanging around in the lobby talking with a retired American businessman who claimed to be an expert on astral projection. The man was calm and assured – he seemed to have an inner peace. He told us that he had been naturally able to astral project as a child, but that the sudden materialisation of his astral self in his parents' bedroom, hovering over their bed, had caused his folks to completely freak out. Later his astral manifestations had come close to causing his wife to have a nervous breakdown. He had decided that it was more important to have a happy home life than embark upon spiritual voyages of self-discovery. However, now that his wife had died and his children were grown and he had retired to his ancestral home of Kerry with a little money, he was finally free to resume his spiritual quest. He had decided to dedicate the remainder of his days to exploring the astral plane. 'Besides,' he said, 'I have nothing else to do now.'

We regarded this man with awe. He was a sage, a soothsayer, a guru. It never occurred to us to ask why he was hanging around the Gresham at the cheerleaders' party. Nor did we wonder why he was so keen to have us visit him individually in his remote bungalow in Kerry where he promised to 'assist' us towards a realisation of our true selves.

At the point where names and addresses were about to be exchanged, a gaggle of giggling cheerleaders suddenly emerged from the party. Our little group of wannabe astral explorers immediately dissolved in pursuit of the cheerleaders.

We didn't get anywhere with the cheerleaders. They had male chaperones so tough they made the Brothers look subtle.

We never got the old man's name or address and he didn't get ours, and we never came across him again.

At least not on this plane of existence anyhow.

★

Fifth and Sixth Year boys could wear their home clothes to school. If they wished, they could smoke in the yard at breaks. Fifth and Sixth Years in Coláiste Mhuire were expected to behave like young adults and would be treated as such by the school.

But you would still be expelled if you were caught speaking English or playing soccer during games. That didn't stop us from expressing ourselves in a form that was guaranteed to outrage the Brothers.

Someone painted a Hitler moustache on the statue of the Virgin Mary that stood inside the front door of the main entrance, arm raised in greeting. The greeting now looked as though the Virgin Mary was giving a Nazi salute. Various Brothers and several students used scouring powder to get rid of the moustache, but their efforts were only partially successful. An investigation was launched, but it proved inconclusive. It took many weeks of work to erase the moustache, but it was still possible to make out a thin outline, especially in the mornings when the light was strongest. A short while later, the moustache reappeared on the Virgin Mary's face. This time, it was accompanied by a Hitler fringe and a swastika on her arm. The swastika was rubbed off, but the other visual atrocities remained for ages, as though the Brothers had given up.

In the yard we held meetings to discuss the growing tensions between the Brothers and some of the pupils. During one lunch break we went to the Garden of Remembrance opposite the school to decide upon a course of action. The Garden of Remembrance was a peaceful spot. There was a long water feature with various flowing fountains and specially made memorial stone works. Established to commemorate the sacrifice of the Rebels of 1916, the gardens now played host to a group of rebellious schoolboys who wanted to indict their teachers.

I argued that vicious perverts like Barreller, Nelly and Canny who ritually abused boys were criminals and should be tried. Thus far, our only way of fighting back was to give some of them nicknames that dehumanised or poked fun at them, but that was no defence.

I thought that we should go to the police.

Everybody agreed that the brutality was unacceptable and unfair, but few wanted to go to the cops about it – that was too drastic. Boys pointed out that there were good Christian Brothers as well as bad. A Brother named Waddy who taught Sixth Class in primary school was held up as an example of a decent man and a good teacher, as was Brother Piggy and several others. But that still left a lot of nasty ones that everyone was afraid of. Some worried that a big scandal would be bad for the school and rebound disastrously on us. We could get a reputation as troublemakers. We might end up so tarnished that we would have difficulty gaining entrance to third-level education or finding jobs.

We voted on it and elected not to go to the cops. Instead we decided that we should seek expert advice.

After one particular beating when Canny hammered a boy for cogging homework, a bunch of us got together one lunchtime and went down to the newspaper offices on Burgh Quay. *The Evening Press* ran a column called 'Ask the Experts' in which various experts answered readers' queries on what seemed like any issue. We figured that the people who wrote 'Ask the Experts' could tell us how to go about getting a Christian Brother put in jail for brutality. After a time, a nice man came downstairs to talk to us. He listened to our tale and he seemed shocked. He explained that we would need corroboration from witnesses and of course a statement from the abused parties. It would be a big help if we could get some responsible adults on board, say a politician or a lawyer. He advised us to talk to our parents. We told him that our parents didn't believe us. He was sympathetic, but he said that there wasn't much else he could do for us. We left the offices somewhat disappointed, but reassured that we had at least been listened to with respect.

Later boys from another class approached some of the lay teachers to complain about the brutality. Apparently, there were discussions between the lay teachers and the Brothers, but I didn't notice much difference. Nelly, Barreller and the Head Brother, Canny, continued to beat boys whenever they felt that they had a reason.

★

In Sixth Year we inherited Jerome, who had remained behind to repeat a year. Jerome was sallow skinned, handsome and intelligent. He was also openly and unapologetically homosexual. He delighted in telling us tales of his sexual conquests – he had had such-and-such a boy from Fifth Class in the downstairs toilets between classes, he had seduced so-and-so from his previous class in the bicycle shed after school one day. I had met actors who were homosexual and had occasionally encountered delicate-looking boys who behaved in an effete way, but I had never met anyone like Jerome. Jerome looked and behaved like a tanned Adonis. There was nothing effete or girly about him. Girls from Scoil Caitríona fancied him. He intrigued and confused us.

Jerome boasted about his lifestyle. After school he usually met his cruising partner, Larry the Taxi Man. Jerome always dumped his schoolbag in the boot of the taxi, and he and Larry spent the rest of the night cruising the city looking for 'chickens', boys Jerome's age or younger. Jerome rarely did homework and nobody ever bothered him about it. The Brothers left

Jerome alone, as though there was some unwritten agreement between them. In return, Jerome rarely took part in any class mischief. He gave the appearance of enjoying all the messing, but he always seemed preoccupied with his life outside school.

I always got the feeling that somebody was protecting Jerome. He seemed to operate on a different level to the rest of us, and he was rarely held accountable for his activities.

At that stage I equated homosexuality with predatory Christian Brothers or with the old male perverts you heard about or occasionally encountered in parks or hanging around outside public toilets. It was a surprise to me that a normal-looking bloke could be gay.

Jerome could be great company. He was funny and he had lots of wicked stories about the Brothers and other teachers. He was bright and articulate and well read. He once read out an essay in a strong, resonant voice. Jerome's essay was actually a short story about a seriously ill older man who was being cared for by a young boy. It was set in Malaysia and evoked an exotic and beguiling atmosphere. Everyone in class was very impressed.

I decided that I didn't like Jerome. Not only was he a preda-tory gay and older and wiser and more experienced in the world than the rest of us, but now he was a writer as well. I was no longer the only writer in the class. My special identity had been undermined.

I began to avoid Jerome whenever I could. I didn't like the way he looked at Cian, my friend. I didn't like the way he encouraged other friends of mine to go out with him. I didn't like the way that he was up for having sex with any of us at any time of the day, either during school or after. I felt uncomfort-able having a predatory gay as a classmate. I didn't know how to handle the situation, so I avoided it.

One day Jerome came into school looking dishevelled and unwashed. He had love bites on his neck and a big bruise on one side of his face. At first he wouldn't talk about it. Later he said that he had done a favour for Larry and that it had been a little more difficult than he had anticipated.

Jerome remained a gentleman to the rest of us. He was good at giving advice and he never, to the best of my knowledge, took advantage of anyone when they were drunk or feeling vulnerable. His maturity didn't stop me disliking him, but we remained on civil terms throughout Sixth Year.

In Sixth Year, Canny left for reasons unknown and a new head was appointed. Hank was tall and grey haired and had an inscrutable expression on his small, pinched face. He walked slowly, without moving his arms. It turned out that Hank had a balance problem. We were told never to approach our new Head Brother from behind or the side. Anything we had to say to Hank should be delivered face to face.

At first we had high hopes for Hank, but he soon showed that he was on a similar wavelength to the nasty Brothers by making use of the leather whenever some boy screwed up his Latin declensions or was caught talking or messing in class. Hank was big on religion. He wanted us to become better Catholics. He worried that kids growing up in a godless place like Dublin would lose their values as well as their belief. Once I nodded off during religion class and he woke me up by slapping me across the head with a dictionary.

That afternoon, he phoned my parents to tell them that I was using drugs. As proof he told them that I had difficulty staying awake in religion class.

I got home to find my parents in uproar. It took nearly an hour before they told me what Hank had said. I denied his accusations and told them that I was going to get an apology from the Head.

The next morning I skipped class and tried to find Hank. I waited outside his office. On several occasions Hank came out and ignored or brushed off my requests for a meeting. I remained seated outside his office for the entire morning. I

stayed there during lunch and for most of the afternoon. I felt
determined and powerful. I was in the right. I didn't care if I
went hungry. Hank had falsely accused me. I wanted him to
apologise and withdraw his allegations. When other Brothers
asked me what I was doing waiting outside the office, I told
them that I had important business with the Head. They left
me alone.

Eventually Hank came up to me to ask me what I wanted. I
told him that I was angry that he had accused me of taking
drugs in religion class when it was untrue. I was angry that he
had told my parents before even discussing it with me.

He thought for a moment. 'OK, I shouldn't have told your
parents,' he said briskly before striding off.

At home afterwards I pleaded with Dad to phone the school
and talk to Hank. At some point Dad made the call. I know that
there was a discussion, but I don't know what was said. The
matter was dropped and never mentioned again.

I felt that I had won a victory. I had taken on the Head
Brother and won. I felt like a superhero. I felt like a lead guitarist in a rock band. I felt as though I had scored a hat trick in
an FA Cup Final.

★

That Easter, the Brothers organised a retreat in our classroom.
They thought some of the Sixth Year boys were beginning to
drift spiritually.

A placid-looking monk arrived. At least we thought he was a
monk. He wore a robe with a cowl. There were prayers all
morning. We were all bored rigid. We noticed that the monk
spent most of his time with his back to us, occupying the area
between two of the front desks. We also noticed that his cowl
was large and hung open and inviting.

We also learned that the retreat had been Hank's idea, his pet project to make us better Catholics. We decided to do something.

At lunchtime we met in the canteen and made a plan. We took chicken legs, half-eaten potatoes, forks, knives, spoons and other bits of food and carried them in our pockets back into the classroom where we were to attend a special afternoon mass.

First, there was a long period of sermons and prayers. The monk took his place with his back to us. Hank and various Brothers recited or read holy texts and led us in prayers.

We surreptitiously passed the various smuggled food items up to the boys at the front. Gently, the items were dropped one at a time and with the utmost delicacy into the monk's cowl. Within ten minutes the cowl bulged with the makings of a full meal, along with cutlery. A final spoonful of jelly had just disappeared into the cowl when the monk was summoned away to the top of the class to perform the mass ceremony.

There was a period of reflective silence before the mass began. Then the monk put up his cowl.

A fork clanged on the altar in front of him, followed by several potatoes, chicken legs and other bits of food. Items continued to drop out of the upraised cowl for several moments. The Brothers stood frozen in horror. The spoonful of jelly fell out last and landed with a *squish* on the altar, which now looked as though it had been the scene of a food fight.

Curiously, there was no expression on the monk's face. He seemed to regard the unsolicited food remnants in his cowl as not totally unexpected.

We remained deadpan in the glare of the Brothers and particularly Hank, who after that incident developed a loathing for us.

★

At some point the Brothers obviously decided that it would be a good thing to hold regular ceilís where the boys from

Coláiste could dance the 'Walls of Limerick' and the like with the girls from Scoil Caitríona, which was at that time Dublin's only Irish-language secondary school for girls.

The ceilís were held at night-time once every few weeks in the big hall in Coláiste Mhuire. They always started off quietly, but grew wilder as the night went on. Some boys met for pints in a pub where the barman didn't ask questions about a boy's age as long as he could pay for the drink.

Others smoked joints before going in. A few took pills or slugged from a bottle of cough medicine called Demerol, a hideous-tasting dark liquid that made you feel that you had just swallowed a raw haddock. I tried it once and threw up in the street. I pretended to smoke dope, but I didn't like it. I didn't really like the taste of drink either, but I quite enjoyed the dizzy confidence that a couple of pints gave me. Before going into the ceilís, we chewed gum. Spearmint was best for getting rid of the smell of stout.

Brothers patrolled the ceilís like piranhas. But even the Brothers couldn't stop boys throwing their partners about during the faster jigs and reels, sometimes deliberately letting go of a twirling girl's hands at an inappropriate moment to send her crashing into a row of other dancers, spilling them like so many human bowling pins. That practice only stopped when some poor girl broke a collarbone.

The ceilís always took place with every light in the hall blazing. The only place you could go with a girl in secret was behind the curtains at the top of the rows of seats, a place where for some reason the Brothers rarely intruded.

I met a girl named Simone at one of the ceilís. She seemed to like me. She told me that she was going to throw a big party and invite some of the boys from Coláiste. I danced with Simone and some of her friends, but I was too shy to ask her out. I figured that something might happen between us at the party.

Simone lived in a nice house somewhere in Dún Laoghaire. The plan was for everyone to bring cider and crisps and stay the night by crashing on the floor or whatever. Simone was blonde and had long legs and I really fancied her. It took me an hour to realise that the boy she was holding hands with was actually her boyfriend and not just a good pal. By that stage, everyone else had paired off.

Halfway through the party Simone's parents came home unexpectedly. It had been a free house, not a legitimate party, so the only thing to do was to scarper. A few of us hid in the coal shed, but we were quickly discovered and turfed out into the street with the others.

There were no late buses and no taxis around. We wandered around looking for shelter. Approximately sixty fifteen- and sixteen-year-old girls and boys ambled around in the freezing cold until we happened upon the Forty Foot, where high walls and rock formations offered a respite from the cold winds. The Forty Foot was a famous swimming spot supposedly for men only. A sign at the entrance proclaimed with unintentional humour, 'Forty Foot Gentlemen Only'. We huddled into corners and behind rocks and tried to keep warm.

We noticed small red glows in the darkness. The red glows belonged to the lit cigarettes of gay men who were all around us, waiting for other gays to arrive for illicit sex. Cars dropped men off while others arrived on foot. We could see nothing in the murk, but we heard rustlings sometimes followed by soft moans. Ironically, Jerome hadn't gone to the party. Some of us speculated that our classmate might be out there in the darkness somewhere.

At first light all the gays had gone, leaving only a trail of cigarette butts.

★

I don't remember whose idea it was to teach Barreller a lesson – it may even have been mine. I don't recall the reason either, but it was probably an accumulation of things that provoked the attempt.

Barreller had been in dreadful temper that week. He had upset quite a few of us with his brutal treatment and sarcastic remarks. On Friday morning a bunch of us placed a large alabaster globe at the top of the geography cabinet, rigged to fall the moment the door was opened. Barreller came in that morning in a fury. He swept through the class, admonishing boys for their attire or for their sloppy homework. Then he went to the cabinet.

Everyone held their breath.

Barreller opened the door and the heavy globe fell out, missing his head by an inch. The globe landed on the wooden floor with a heavy boom. It did not bounce or move. The globe was so heavy that it made a deep indentation in the wooden floorboards, like a bomb crater.

Barreller stared in disbelief at the object that had just missed his head, and then he looked accusingly at us. He knew what had just happened. The class had attempted to bump him off or at the very least severely injure him. He walked out of the class and slammed the door.

Immediately, I felt guilty. I felt sorry that we had humiliated the man who now somehow seemed like a creature of flesh and blood with human feelings instead of a monster.

In silence, some of us picked up the globe and put it back in the cabinet. This time, we placed it on the bottom shelf.

★

The end came one morning about three months before we took our final exams, the Leaving Cert.

For some reason, perhaps because we were expecting a class with Matty, our easy-going Irish-language teacher, we decided to switch all the desks around to face the wall behind, upon which we drew a rough blackboard. We obscured the real blackboard with the coat racks.

Then we sat down in our back-to-front classroom, pretending to be deep in study. But Matty was sick, and Hank arrived as his replacement. Hank lost his balance momentarily on walking into the back-to-front class. When he had finished wobbling, he told us to take our bags and get out of the school. He was expelling the lot of us and he wasn't prepared to discuss it.

Slowly, we got our bags and coats and left the class. Then we filed down the stairs in silence and left the school building.

Outside on the street, we were deeply shocked. I felt a mixture of elation and terror. I was out of the school for good, but I had been expelled. There would be consequences. My life could be ruined. I was really in trouble now.

After a brief discussion, we decided to go to the Del Rio Restaurant to talk things over and come up with a plan. Some boys went home, but most of us walked to Abbey Street and bought pots of tea in the Del Rio, which was directly opposite the Abbey Theatre. As we talked I kept a lookout for my dad, who sometimes dropped into the Del Rio to buy tea or coffee or to have a private chat with an actor.

We decided that the expulsion had been coming for a long time. We could do nothing except go home and tell our parents. Our camaraderie remained intact. There were no accusations of blame. We worried about what our parents would say, but we were also troubled that the school would not allow us to sit the finals.

I went home to Howth on the bus. There was no little red bus for some reason so I phoned Dad from the call box outside the library. He drove down to collect me. I got into the car and he drove up the hill. We travelled in silence. Nearing home, I began to say something, but Dad held up his hand. 'Don't say another word,' he said.

Mother gave me a lecture. I don't remember what she said.

I must have closed down from shame and embarrassment. I said I was sorry. I told them that the school was a brutal place and we had reacted with mischief because we had been badly treated. My parents didn't buy that. I was sent to my room.

Following representations from outraged and disgusted parents, the school allowed seven or eight boys to return to classes. However, the Brothers regarded myself and several others as the ringleaders of the back-to-front classroom stunt as well as instigators of many other school atrocities. They refused to allow the rest of us back into the classroom, but they could not prevent us sitting our finals in the school hall.

I was told to go to my room and study hard.

The newspapers rang the next morning. I talked to a reporter for a few moments and refused to allow my name to be given. I told the reporter that the boys had been at loggerheads with the school authorities. I don't know where I got loggerheads from or why I used it – the word just popped out.

That evening the front page of the evening paper contained a report about a final-year class being expelled from Dublin's prestigious Irish-language school. The newspaper quoted an unnamed pupil to the effect that the class had been at 'loggerheads' with the school authorities for some time. The headline read 'Loggerheads'.

Mortified yet oddly exhilarated as well, I went to my room and studied harder. Perhaps for the first time in my life I really learned from my schoolbooks. I figured that studying at home was a far better way to acquire knowledge than sitting in a dank classroom in Coláiste Mhuire.

A few months later we sat the final exams. I enjoyed the English exam so much that I lost track of time and finished an hour early. As I was waiting outside for the others, a Brother named Dunbar came up and asked why I had left early. I explained that I had got the time wrong. Dunbar sneered at me, 'Mac Anna, you're well and truly up the Swanee now.'

When the exams were finished the seventeen of us went out into the world. Some went to college, others took jobs or left the country. I qualified for an Arts degree at UCD.

We made valiant attempts to keep what remained of the class together. For many months we met once a week in the upstairs lounge of a city-centre pub, but within a year, the meetings stopped. Some of the boys stayed friends, but I gradually drifted away from my former classmates.

9

Dancing in the Broom Closet

Going to college was the obvious thing for me to do. I didn't know how to get the things I wanted from my life and I didn't want to take a plunge into the real world of work – there weren't that many jobs around anyway. After an uneventful first year at UCD (where I was supposed to be studying English and History), I decided to go to London for the summer because it seemed like everyone I knew in UCD had been in London the summer before.

Guys boasted of the great bands they'd seen and the fantastic sex they'd had with London girls. London girls were wild things. The guys also came back with enough dosh to get them through a college year.

I couldn't wait to get there.

A friend from Howth had been in London the previous summer and gave me the phone number of Janet, a landlady who rented cheap accommodation to students.

My pal Big D and I took the ferry to Holyhead in Wales. The ferry was packed with students and navvies going back to the sites. The sea was rough and people slithered back and forth along wet decks.

'The bathrooms are like a jeweller's shop,' Big D said. 'People keep leaving their rings in there.'

It was a depressing trip, but I was upbeat because I was getting away from home and Ireland and everything I had known. It was also my first time abroad on my own. I felt totally free.

We caught a smelly, overcrowded train from Holyhead to Euston. The seats were cramped, but I was still happy and excited. I might not come back to Dublin, I thought. There was every chance that I could find my destiny in London.

We arrived at Euston at eight in the morning, bleary eyed. I phoned Janet the Landlady and she gave us directions to her place in Finchley in North London.

Janet was a tall, aristocratic Jewish woman in her thirties. She lived with her small daughter in a two-bedroom apartment above a pub called The Swan and Pyramid. She had a back bedroom she could let us have. The bedroom was basically a box room with bunks and a single bed. I took the single bed. Big D took one of the bunk beds. The other bunk bed was already taken by Robbie, a black Londoner with a neat afro.

The next day I started a job as a labourer on a building site. My job was to carry stuff.

Everyone called me Paddy. After a few hours a couple of brickies asked me my real name. Ferdia, I told them. They looked at each other and went back to calling me Paddy.

The worst part of my new job was trying to haul acros (heavy iron poles that were used to prop up ceilings while building work continued) and I tried to find a different job on site. I got talking to the foreman, a chap from Clare who sported a handlebar moustache that made him look like a Battle of Britain Spitfire pilot. He told me that he had known my father.

He had been part of a drama group that had performed an O'Casey at an amateur drama festival that my father had adjudicated. His group had come last. He had never gotten over the disappointment. He told me that if I kept my nose clean and kept toting acros, there might be a plasterer's job going in about a year's time.

One day a crane operator lost control of a load of steel girders. The load swung wildly as girders dropped hundreds of feet to the ground. Everywhere you looked people ran for cover.

Except me. I stood watching the load of girders swing crazily as though I was at a carnival entertainment. Girders rained down, demolishing a wall and clanging off tractors. One narrowly missed a portakabin. Another girder embedded itself in the earth, sticking up like a thrown javelin. Eventually an old Dublin navvy pulled me into a ditch. Nobody got hurt, but several walls were destroyed. Once the crisis was past, a bunch of labourers, including me, were detailed to gather the fallen girders.

Afterwards the crane driver was fired for being drunk. I heard later that he was reinstated the following week after the foreman got him to swear on the Bible that he would never again visit the pub at lunchtime.

★

One evening towards the end of my first week I came home wrecked. Unable to focus on the TV and too tired to chat to Big D or the others, I drank a cup of tea and went straight to bed.

Within what seemed like a few moments after dropping off I was awakened by noises. I squinted in the dark room. Standing above me was a naked woman. She was a big girl with enormous, firm breasts and long, dark, wavy hair. She was looking down at me with a curious expression on her face, like she was looking at a litter of pups trying to work out which one to choose. 'You sure he's asleep, then? 'E don't look bleedin' asleep to me.'

'Don't worry 'bout 'im, dahlin. 'E's out cold,' a man's voice said. 'Now come on.'

The naked woman disappeared from my squinting eye line. I reckoned I must have been dreaming.

A few moments later I heard rustling noises followed by creaking bedsprings. Then came smooching noises along with sounds of slobbering. There was a sudden sharp intake of breath, followed by momentary silence.

Then she started to scream and I knew I wasn't in a dream.

She yelled out what she wanted him to do to her and how fast she wanted him to do it. She called him sweet names and then abused him. She wanted it harder and faster. She wanted it now, now, now, NOW…

'Go on Robbie, Go on, go on, go on… Robbie you fucker…'

After a while I slowly turned around to watch the action. I was wide awake and, besides, there was nothing else to do.

They were fucking on the bottom bunk. She was underneath him with her pale legs wedged into the underside of the bunk above. She was palely luminous in the light from the street-lights. His dark shape was arched above her with his arms splayed, holding on to the sides of the bed as he thrust repeatedly into her.

At times, the writhing bodies in the peculiar light made it seem like she was making love to her own shadow.

I was still basically a virgin. I had only been intimate with two girls and neither for very long. Neither had screamed, 'Fuck me faster, you fucker.'

The springs screeched. The bunks bounced up and down on the wooden floor. The whole room seemed to be shaking. She yelled like a maniac. His grunts grew louder with each thrust. The pair became so engrossed in their lovemaking that I could have got out of bed, dressed, pulled up a chair to within inches of their bodies to study and take notes and they would not have noticed.

Watching them, I became aroused. This was exactly the kind of experience I had come to London to find – except that I was in bed alone while others were having the fun. I wanted to meet a London girl who yelled like that because it sounded so thrilling. I wondered if there was a special trick that made women carry on like that. If I studied Robbie's technique closely, perhaps I would pick up a few tips. He didn't seem to be doing anything special or different – just going in and out really fast, stopping for a bit and then going in and out really fast again. Maybe he was performing some secret sex trick in the dark that I couldn't see.

Eventually, the couple finished. Robbie flopped down on top of her, breathing heavily. She gasped that it was the best it had ever been.

I rolled over and thought about what I had seen. I was glad that I was in London. I couldn't imagine an Irish girl carrying on like that or even making love with her boyfriend while there was someone else in the room. Maybe I had been hanging around with the wrong sort of girls. In Ireland I had once spent weeks nurturing and flattering and paying attention to the every whim of a girl I had met at a tennis-club dance. I had ended up with a swift peck on the lips followed by the traditional kiss-off, 'Listen, you're a nice guy, but…'

I decided that I would remain in London at the end of the summer and learn about what it was like to live in a healthy society. I didn't care about college anymore. College was irrelevant to real life.

I was on the verge of dropping off when they started again.

This time she yelled twice as loudly while Robbie grunted louder and faster. The bedsprings again went mental. Apparently, this time was even better for her than the first.

When they got into it for the third time I decided that I had had enough. I climbed out of bed, pulled on my shirt and trousers and left the room without hearing the couple break rhythm for a second.

In the living room all the lights were blazing. The instant I entered, Janet, Big D and several others fell about laughing and gave me a round of applause. They had been placing bets on how long I would last before having to get out. Janet had won a tenner. We could still hear Robbie's girlfriend shouting the roof off. 'They do go on a bit, don't they?' Janet said.

★

After a couple of weeks Big D went home to take up a job offer. Rob the Lover moved out and was replaced by a quiet Cockney named Peter. Robbie's friend, Trevor, moved in as well. Peter became infatuated with the barmaid from the pub downstairs and for days agonised about asking her out. Finally, one night he convinced us to accompany him from for moral support. We stood at the bar while he tried to catch her eye. He was going to give up a couple of times, but we persuaded him to give it a chance. Finally he ordered drinks and asked her out almost in the same breath. The barmaid said yes. Later it turned out that she had fancied him the moment she first saw him. The next night I came home to find Peter and the barmaid entwined in each other's arms in the lower bunk bed.

Emboldened by Peter's example, I was determined to find a girlfriend.

A couple of nights later I sat down next to an attractive girl at a Kilburn and the High Roads gig in the Torrington Arms just down the road. After a while I leaned over and as smoothly as I could I asked the girl if she wanted a drink. She nodded and said she'd have a Guinness. After the gig we got talking. She was from Canada. Her name was Joan. We clicked. She said goodnight to her friends and I walked her to her Tube stop. Outside a chipper, we kissed. It was a clumsy kiss, but it got us both excited. I shyly asked her to come back to Janet's. 'OK,' she said, so we walked, hand in hand, back to the house. Joan didn't talk much so I gabbled on about Dublin and rock music. There was nobody in Janet's living room, so I led her straight to the bedroom. Nobody in the bedroom either. Brilliant. I was away. We kissed again and took off our clothes. I kept thinking that this was too easy. There was bound to be a catch. I fetched the packet of condoms from my case, the packet I had bought on my first day in London. We didn't speak. She helped me get the condom on. It took a while and the situation made us laugh.

Our lovemaking was awkward, as though we were waiting for someone to hand us a sex manual. I had the distinct feeling that I was not the only one who was saying goodbye to virginity. I enjoyed it, but it was confusing. I couldn't understand why she wasn't yelling the roof off like Robbie's girlfriend. Perhaps she wasn't enjoying it. Maybe I was doing something wrong. I tried going fast, then stopping suddenly for a bit, then taking off like Speedy Gonzalez again. It got me pretty excited, but I couldn't tell how she felt about it. It felt strange to be wearing a condom. At times I felt like my cock was being strangled. When I finally came I made an involuntary gasp – and she immediately gave an answering gasp. Either we had achieved nirvana at the same moment or else she was trying to make me feel good.

After she fell asleep I tossed around all night, unable to get comfortable in the narrow bed. In the morning we made love again – this time it was better. I felt as though I almost knew what I was doing. Certainly it was easier to get the condom on, but that may have been because of the morning light, which meant that I could actually see where I was aiming. I wondered if sex was always like this – self-conscious, confusing and performed to a rhythm that was punctuated by squelching sounds.

I found out that Peter had spent the night at the barmaid's and Trevor had graciously elected to sleep on the sofa once he had realised that I had female company.

After breakfast I walked Joan to the local Tube, where she asked for my phone number. Flattered, I wrote it down for her but, intoxicated by my conquest, I deliberately juggled up the numbers. Having successfully lost my virginity, I was now certain to click with dozens of other girls. I kissed her goodbye, but she stayed put.

She looked at me over her glasses. 'Don't you want my number?'

Embarrassed, I wrote down her number on a piece of paper. Once she had disappeared into the Tube station I scrunched the piece of paper up and tossed it into a bin. I walked back to Janet's feeling like James Bond. Love them and leave them.

Later I came to my senses. It dawned on me that I had tossed away my first London girlfriend. I felt like a complete fool.

★

At weekends I hung around with my old school pal Marvo, who had been in London for a year. As far as I was concerned, Marvo was the King of London. He dressed well, he always had a mischievous look on his face, plus he had a job, money and his own apartment. He turned every night into an adventure. I was impressed by his newly acquired London sayings. He said 'nice one' about virtually everything that happened, good as well as bad. 'This is what we find' was also used as a reaction to virtually any occurrence. Nothing seemed to put him off or dampen his enthusiasm. He was into having fun as often and for as long as possible.

I became friends with Marvo's friend Joey, a London-Irish lad the same age as me. Joey was as passionate about rock music as I was and we discovered a pub called the Flowerpot that played hard rock albums over a huge sound system. Joey liked Budgie, Led Zeppelin and Deep Purple. I was still into Thin Lizzy and The Groundhogs, as well as weird prog-rock groups like Audience and Gnidrolog. We both liked Jethro Tull.

Joey was quite shy and his shyness seemed to increase daily. I always had to call to his house in Wood Green to get him to come out. His mother – a quiet-spoken, elegant Donegal woman – took me aside to ask me to continue calling for Joey. She was worried that he was so shy that he would one day refuse to leave the house altogether. I made the mistake of telling Joey what his mother had said. Joey got mad at his mother and his mother got mad at me.

One night Marvo and Joey and I plus several others went drinking in the West End. We saw a band called Zzebra, drank lots of pints and smoked joints. We took tabs of acid as well, though I have no memory of who brought them or why we decided to drop them. We ended up rolling about in Soho, completely out of our heads. Whenever anyone spoke I saw multicoloured letters of the alphabet cascading from their mouths.

Somehow we made it back to Janet's apartment, where we sat around drinking coffee and playing the two record albums that someone in the apartment owned at the time – *Sheet Music* by 10cc and *Deep Purple in Concert with the Royal Philharmonic Orchestra.*

I couldn't talk. I lay down and tripped to the music.

Eventually the others fell asleep, but I stayed awake all night listening to side two of *Sheet Music.* The record player had stuck on automatic so the same side kept playing over and over again. I was too exhausted to get up and switch it off.

While I was in London my family at home did not exist. They weren't even a memory. College did not exist. In London there was only my every waking moment of trying to discover new and exciting experiences, a hyper search for kicks. I entered into my new life with fervour. I drank, I smoked and I puffed on joints whenever someone had dope. Somehow, the summer frittered away. I never found another girlfriend, but in many ways I was too busy getting trashed to worry about it.

For Trevor's birthday we threw a big party in Janet's. We invited girls but none showed up, except for the barmaid, who left early saying she had to go to her mother's. When the man from next door knocked on the door to complain about the noise, Janet told him to loosen up and tugged on the belt of his nightgown. Then Janet closed the front door and we all danced to Trevor's Uriah Heep album.

After Janet went to bed Trevor produced a small keyboard and an amplifier. He played along to 'Look at Yourself'. By four in the morning even Janet had had enough. She came out of her room in a fury and threw us all out. I went back to Trevor's parents' house and slept on his father's collapsible military bed.

In the morning, hung over and contrite, I went back to Janet's. She refused to let me back in except to gather my stuff and get out. Sorrowfully, I went into the bedroom and packed my gear.

I was about to leave the apartment when the phone rang. Janet answered it. She looked taken aback. 'It's your father. He wants to know when you're coming home.'

★

The following summer six of us arrived in London. Our accommodation had fallen through, so we all crashed on Marvo's floor for a week. We were huddled together on the King of London's floorboards like guinea pigs in someone's laboratory.

We found a house to rent in Tottenham and moved in. I got a job with Thorn's, a catering company that delivered chairs, tables and cutlery all over London and sometimes as far as

Oxford. The Cockneys who worked there called what they did 'Thornicatering'.

On my first morning on the job I got a lift to the depot with the owner in his Rolls Royce. The owner was an elderly, fat Cockney with a face that seemed incapable of showing expression. He told me that I could have a car like his one day if I worked hard and kept an eye open for good opportunities.

At the end of the first week Brosh, a young Londoner who had been avoiding me all week, came up to me. 'You live in Dublin, do yer?'

I told him that I did. I could tell by his tone and manner that he was trying to provoke a rise out of me. 'A lot of stupid people live in that place, don't they?' he said.

I didn't know what to say to that. It seemed to me that any answer I gave would be the wrong one. I didn't want to get into a ruckus in my first week on the job, but I couldn't let him walk on me. I said that stupid people lived everywhere. He stared into my eyes for a hard moment. I thought he was about to start swinging in front of all our colleagues. Then he relaxed, and he walked away. 'Dublin has lots of really stupid people,' he shouted back. I said nothing.

A few days later I discovered that he was second-generation Irish – his parents were from Dublin. I got on OK with him after that.

I fancied Fiona, a petite blonde who shared the house in Tottenham. I had watched her drive around UCD on her Yamaha 50 without a helmet. I thought she looked like a young Brigitte Bardot. I had been too timid to talk to her in UCD. In London I figured I stood a better chance, possibly because we were living in the same house. Fiona got a job as a barmaid at the Mitre pub so I started going down for a drink after work. I couldn't tell if she was interested in me or not. I was rarely alone with her for long enough to find out – some of the others from the house also decided to gather there after work.

One night coming home from the Mitre a bit drunk, I got

into a minor scrap with two black guys at the corner of our road. Initially, the altercation came about because I was clumsy and bumped into them while trying to pass them on the footpath. There was a bit of shoving and I dropped the bottle of beer I had been drinking. Trying to pick up the broken glass, I accidentally cut my hand. In my drunkenness I saw an opportunity. I had been in a fight. There had been a bottle. The fight had happened because someone said something about Fiona. I walked back to the house. From time to time I dabbed a little blood from my hand on my head. I thought it might look more dramatic. It worked.

The girl who opened the door saw my face and immediately fainted. I looked like something from *The Texas Chainsaw Massacre*. Other housemates grabbed me and brought me into the front room to clean me up. Someone put a plaster on my hand. Nobody could figure out why there was so much blood on my face but no cut. I told them a dramatic story about getting in a fight with two guys on my way home. Most believed me, but a couple of the male housemates were suspicious.

The next day the word was out. At work guys wanted to help me track down the ones who'd bottled me. The barman in the Mitre said he'd bar the guys and to tell him immediately if I ever saw them come into the pub. I tried to play it all down, but it had gone too far. I felt like I had told my own version of my mother's Spanish Armada story. Deep inside I was mortified, but I stuck to my story because I was too embarrassed to admit that I had spoofed it up to make myself appear heroic.

There was tension in the house. I wasn't getting along with a couple of the guys who had been dubious about my fight story. In the Mitre a couple of weeks later I got into a very public row with one of the guys and I ended up punching him. Later I apologised and the two of us eventually became good friends, but for a while I felt like the last gunslinger in town. I became paranoid that everyone was going to want to take a pop at me. Was I now hanging around with bad company? Or had I become the bad company that mothers warned their kids about?

A few weeks later we threw a party in the house. People from the Mitre came back, including a bunch of locals we had befriended, and several of my 'Thornicaterer' workmates. Somehow I ended up in a broom closet with Fiona. We kissed and remained there until I shifted my foot and accidentally kicked the closet door down. It glided gracefully into the front room like a kite before settling gently on the floor, whereupon everyone stopped dancing to have a good gawk at the two eejits who were cuddling in the broom closet.

Afterwards Fiona and I started going out together. She moved out of the upstairs bedroom that she was sharing with two other girls and we occupied the sofa in the front room. She was my first serious girlfriend and the first woman I truly loved.

When the lease for the house in Tottenham ended, some people went home while Fiona and myself and several others moved into a squat down the road. Fiona got a job in Central London, working for the tourist board. Joey and I got jobs in a bakery in Wood Green.

On Fiona's birthday, as a surprise, I bought a large cream-filled birthday cake in a Greek bakery near where I worked. I brought it home on the Tube, hoping that nobody would bump into it and smudge the cream letters that spelled 'Happy Birthday Fiona'. I walked through sodden streets in the rain and eventually got back to the house, stashed the cake in the fridge and rushed upstairs to our bedroom. I opened the door and found Fiona asleep in bed with flames devouring the bedside table and the bedclothes around her. I rushed to the window and opened it. Somehow I managed to haul the table over and push it out the open window. I didn't even look to see if there was anyone below. Then I grabbed the pillows and bedclothes and tossed them out as well.

Fiona woke up and gave me a dreamy smile. 'Hi there,' she said. 'Welcome home.'

She had no idea of what had just happened.

She had gone for drinks after work, come home exhausted and decided to take a nap. Before conking out she had lit the candle on the bedside table. Obviously the candle had toppled over when she was asleep and set fire to the bedclothes. I had arrived home just in time.

I worked in the bakery for a couple of months. I was due back in college in October, but I had no real interest in going. Then again, I didn't want to stay in London doing shift work in a bakery for the rest of my days. Most of the time I didn't even work alongside Joey anymore. Fiona wasn't interested in going back to college. She wanted to remain in London for a few months to save money, but I was restless.

My parents were trying to contact me. It was time to go home. I liked having no responsibilities. I liked being free. College meant that I had something to come back to. Despite all my talk about living in London and the freedom and opportunities that there were away from Ireland, deep inside I must have wanted to come home to finish my course.

Eventually my sense of self-preservation kicked in and I decided to go back home.

Fiona had to work on my last day in London so I arranged to visit Joey to say goodbye. By this stage, I had amassed quite a collection of LPs to bring home. We spent the morning and afternoon in his bedroom, drinking cider and playing records. He played a side of Budgie or Deep Purple. Then I got to put on a side of my choice. We talked and drank and listened. We made plans. He would quit the bakery and come to Dublin next summer. We would learn instruments and form a band. We would save our money and head for Greece.

When it was time for me to go, Joey accompanied me to the train station. We said goodbye and I got on the train and left London. We promised to keep in touch and write, but we never did.

★

After a long, tedious journey by train and ferry, I arrived back in Howth train station at around seven on a rosy morning. The air was crisp and scraped the inside of my throat and nostrils. I felt as though I had woken up from a deep dream about London. I caught the first little red bus up the hill.

I got off the bus and carried my bags the few yards to my home. I met Dad at the bottom of the driveway putting out bins. He looked surprised, as though he had never expected to see me again. 'Oh,' he said. 'Well, you're back. You'd better talk to your mother.'

He turned around and walked up the driveway, and after a moment I followed.

10

UCD, 1976 (Johnny Jurex)

I am a third-year arts student, studying English and History. I am very tall, skinny and mopey with long, dark and sometimes greasy hair. I wear denims most of the time. I like cheesecloth shirts and drainpipe jeans. Occasionally I remember to wash my hair.

I lust after most of the good-looking girls on campus, but I am too shy to do anything about it – unless I am drunk. I have the occasional fling but nothing serious, so mostly I am single and frustrated. I drink too much at night and sometimes during the day. Occasionally I smoke dope, but I don't care for it much – it makes me feel like my hair is trying to strangle me. On a bad night, it feels like other people's hair is trying to strangle me.

I am always in a hurry to do something, but I am not always sure of what it is that I want to do. I want to be a writer, but I am usually in such a rush that I can never find the time to write.

UCD is a dull campus. The Arts Block is a series of dreary concrete chambers, filled with endless dark corridors and face-less students.

I don't care for most of the professors. The ones in the Department of English are a smug lot – in lectures they give the impression that they are superior to the writers we are studying. To listen to some of them, you could be mistaken for believing that literary criticism is the true essence of artistic endeavour.

So I don't go to lectures much. I avoid tutorials whenever possible as well. If I had my way, I would abolish all lectures and tutorials and just ask people to read the books. That's what I do. I just read the books on the course and take my chances in the exams. It seems to be working. I have made it to my final year. Just.

I knock around with some of the radical socialists, though I don't share their views. I don't subscribe to any political creed. However, I admit to having a soft spot for anarchism. This is because of a history book, *Anarchism,* by George Woodcock, which is filled with eccentric and often dangerous characters like Bakhunin, whose central philosophy is that in order to create a good and just society, you first had to destroy the one that exists. Walking around the grim corridors of UCD, I can relate to that.

I write an occasional column for the student rag under the pen name Luigi 'Knuckles' Bombalini, Professor of English at the University of Naples. I invent a new kind of poetry, Mafia Gangster Verse. Here's a sample: 'Ode to Mugsy'.

O Mugsy.
Why didya
havta go
and do it?
You shouldn'ta
Mugsy
Cos now
You is
No more.

It doesn't catch on.

I am bored. I would like to quit and get a real job, but I am scared of what my folks would say. I am also a bit intimidated by the real world. It seems there are no jobs, just a desert of unemployment. It's a very difficult time for graduates and many of my friends plan to emigrate to England or the US. Some are heading for Germany. Anywhere, really, except Ireland.

I also want to stay and finish my degree. I am nearly there with just a few months to go. I don't know what I want to do when I finish. Perhaps I'll write, but maybe not yet. I want to do a bit of living first. I want to have fun.

On campus there is a small buzz about punk. The Sex Pistols are in the news for mouthing obscenities on a live chat show in England. John Peel is playing songs by The Damned and The Buzzcocks. Arguments abound in the Belfield Bar and the canteen between those who like the Pistols and the Pink Floyd and Rolling Stones fans who say that the 'new music' is rubbish.

I love the new music. I love its energy and its do-it-yourself attitude. I buy records by The Ramones and Blondie and most of the new American bands, the so-called 'blank generation'. I buy my first punk singles, 'Neat, Neat, Neat' by The Damned and 'White Riot' by The Clash. I love the way the outrage over punk's lack of musical ability or reverence shows up the rock establishment as reactionary old dorks.

I decide to form a punk rock band for Rag Week to send up the whole thing. We'll play a gig and write our own songs. It'll be a laugh.

I want to give the college authorities a bit of a scare. I want to see what it's like to be in a band. Besides, there's this girl I fancy called Mary. She is tall and dark and comes from Cork. She is good looking with a soft voice and a cute smile and is almost as tall as me. I know some of her friends and have occasionally spoken to Mary herself, but I am too chicken to ask her out. I haven't even told any of my friends that I fancy her.

I figure that she will fancy me once I'm in a band. Even if it's only a doss band.

I don't dwell on the fact that I can't play an instrument or sing. This is the time of punk. You can do anything you want. In my band, nobody should be able to play an instrument. The aim is to take the piss out of the whole punk thing.

I strut into the Students' Union and inform the Rag Week Committee guy that I've got a punk band.

'Great,' he says. 'What are you called?'

'Johnny Jurex and the Punk Pistols,' I say, having plucked the name from somewhere inside my head.

He books us for a lunchtime gig in the Aula Max on Tuesday – four days' time. I convince my friend McClelland to join the band. He thinks the name is wild.

'I'll be Johnny Jurex and you can be Jimmy Jurex. We've got a gig in the Aula Max.'

McClelland looks concerned, 'We do? Already! What about instruments?'

'I'll get the instruments and the Students' Union is getting us a PA.'

'Great, what are we going to sing?'

'We'll write our own songs.'

'Are we not going to rehearse?'

'No!'

I tell him that I've already got a song. It's called 'Fuck Bill Grundy'.

'How does it go?'

'Fuck Bill Grundy. Fuck Bill Grundy. Fuck Bill Grundy. Fuck Bill Grundy.'

'Is that all?' McClelland says. 'It's a bit short.'

'That's the whole point. No song is longer than one minute.'

'We'll need a lot of songs,' McClelland says.

I concede that he has a point. We head to the bar and write another song. We come up with 'Anarchy in Belfield' and sing the first verse. 'Anarchy in Belfield. Anarchy in Belfield. Anarchy in Belfield. Anarchy in Belfield. Kick down the library door. Puke and vomit on the library floor. Anarchy in Belfield.'

I am a guy in a hurry. I have no time to waste on rehearsals. There are posters to draw. Band members to recruit.

We put the word out: 'Punk Band starting. No previous experience necessary.'

McClelland persuades his pal Sherlock to play drums. The deal is no rehearsals and all songs are to be made up on the spot.

'Brilliant,' Sherlock says. 'We'll be like that band from Czechoslovakia, The Plastic People of the Universe.' Sherlock is big into obscure Eastern European rock.

'No we won't,' I tell him. 'We'll be an Irish punk band.'

'Fair enough so,' Sherlock says.

We get no replies to our ads, but we convince a student activist, a Che Guevara lookalike named Shay, to join. Shay has a two-string violin that he can't play. Perfect.

A med student named Chris owns a set of uilleann pipes and is keen to join. Only trouble is that he can play. Still, we need band members. We tell Chris he can join as long as he plays the pipes out of tune.

Delighted, Chris agrees.

I run into Mary in the Belfield canteen. I pluck up the courage and ask her to be in the band. 'Sounds like a bit of craic,' she says. She agrees as long as she doesn't have to miss any lectures.

'It's a lunchtime gig,' I tell her. 'No rehearsals.'

'What do I have to do?'

'We'll give you a guitar, just strum it as fast as you can.'

'Grand,' she says. 'I'm in.'

We put up posters. Spread the word. Robert, my friend from Howth, organises a female backing chorus. 'You have to have chick singers,' he says. 'I'll bring Anne and Mairead and Geraldine.' Robert appoints himself unofficial master of ceremonies as well as president of the fan club.

Tuesday arrives. That morning I am so excited I can barely speak. I throw myself into a whirl of mad activity. I wear black jeans and a black shirt. I walk around the campus in cheap black sunglasses. For some reason I buy four cans of shaving foam – I figure they might come in handy for something.

The band meets backstage and goes over the set. We have twelve songs. Not enough. We write another couple backstage.

I announce that everyone should paint their faces white. We want people to 'notice' us, I tell them. We want people to know they have been to a 'punk gig'.

We try painting our faces with the shaving foam but it goes up our noses and drips onto people's clothes. The female backing chorus produce make-up. Soon we are all going around white faced like characters from Bob Dylan's *Rolling Thunder Review*. Sherlock says we look like we have stepped out of a medieval play.

Admission is twenty pence. Five minutes after the doors open, the place is heaving. The crowd expects a real band. They think they're going to see the Irish Sex Pistols. Backstage, we are nervous. This is supposed to be a lark, but now it feels too much like a real event. Maybe we should have rehearsed. Perhaps we should have got real musicians to help out. What have I got myself into? I can't relax, though I am careful not to let on.

I smile at Mary, but she is busy messing with her friends, who are arranging her hair.

I look around at all the white faces and figure that this is what it is like to be in a real band. The rumble of the crowd outside. The feel of a cool guitar in your hands. Someone passing around a bottle of wine. Tingling expectation in your blood. A girl that you fancy alongside.

We can't play a note, but surely that's the whole point. The crowd will get it, won't they?

Sherlock looks like he's going to throw up. McClelland looks tense. 'They're going to throw us in the lake,' he says.

Charlie McNally, President of the Students' Union, announces us. Huge applause and raucous cheering. Charlie has brought his 'harp'. He wants to jam with us.

'OK,' we say. 'Just don't play anything we know.'

We take the stage. The crowd erupts. McClelland and I hold electric guitars. We plug in. Power surges though the guitars. As I touch the strings, the amp crackles and gurgles. Reality suddenly bites hard. I am petrified. I wish I knew how to play something. Anything. Even one song. Even 'Two Little Boys Had Two Little Toys'. How are we going to get away with this?

We have arranged a big theatrical opening. Lanky Mick walks slowly on stage and lies down in front of Sherlock's drum kit – a snare drum plus a set of overturned dustbins. Mick holds a fishing rod atop of which is perched a cymbal for Sherlock's drums.

We launch into 'Fuck Bill Grundy'. The chorus is the same as the verse. We just yell out the words and take aim. We sound like a plane wreck. The crowd loves it. We play 'Anarchy in Belfield'. Some people sing along. Others just look perplexed.

Halfway through, Charlie McNally joins us on stage unin-vited and adds to the cacophony by blowing his harmonica into a mike. The place goes insane. People invade the stage. We spend as much time repelling invaders as we do taking aim at our instruments.

Towards the end, some eejit sprays a fire hose at the stage, nearly frying us all. 'Bring that bloke down here,' Che Guevara says. 'We want to puke on him.'

The gig ends in noise and confusion, but also wild applause and cheering, including demands for an encore.

We narrowly escape being thrown in the lake and escape to the bar where we drink up all the twenty-pence admission fees. Mary gives me a peck on the cheek and goes off with her boyfriend. Boyfriend? I should have guessed. A big rugger-bugger in a cardigan. My heart plunges, but not for long. We get drunk and sing 'Fuck Bill Grundy'.

Some guy comes up to McClelland and asks us when the first record is coming out. 'Soon,' McClelland tells him and the guy goes off, delighted.

The next day, the others go about their studies. Rag Week ends and college goes back to normal. But my blood is still tingling – I can't wait to do it all again. This time I want to do it for real.

★

The only punk gigs in town are at Moran's Hotel, so I start going there. I dress in black. I cut my shoulder-length hair to just below my ears.

I see gigs by The Boomtown Rats, The Vipers and The Radiators from Space. The Vipers are cool and angry and have some great songs. The Radiators have neat harmonies and the lead singer tosses himself around the stage like a rag doll. The Rats are basically a Dublin version of Dr Feelgood – I have seen them lots of times over the past few years. Now they appeal to punks as well because of Bob Geldof's in-your-face attitude. I thought to myself, if those guys can do it…

One night I drag McClelland and Sherlock along to Moran's. The Rats are playing. During a new song called 'Drive on Damo' (about their van driver), two of them go offstage and re-emerge as the two halves of a pantomime horse. The horse splits in two and everyone cracks up. Not very punk, but funny all the same. Geldof tells the crowd that if they don't like the horse they can 'fuck off'. He gets a huge cheer.

McClelland and Sherlock are amused by all the punks wearing safety pins and pink hair and, as McClelland put it, 'trousers that seemed to have been cast off by some Scottish lowlands regiment'.

I am in punk heaven. It's not just the music, it's the feeling that you can do anything. All you need is the guts to take a risk.

By the time the gig finishes I am almost delirious with

enthusiasm. On the street outside I go on a rant about The Ramones and Blondie and punk rock and the important things that are happening in music today. McClelland and Sherlock humour me. I tell them that this is 'my music, urban music'. 'I'm a city man,' I announce. 'This is my culture.'

They look at me with big, compassionate eyes. I become so intoxicated by my passion for the new music that I start to shout. It is a quiet Saturday night, even in Abbey Street there are no crowds and I keep on making my loud speech.

I spy a number thirty-one bus for Howth pulling out. My bus. I run after it, still shouting. Catching up with the bus, I grab the rail and swing myself aboard. Turning, I wave back to McClelland and Sherlock, who are standing there looking at me like they are watching the last speech of a condemned man.

They give me long, sad waves goodbye.

11

The Birth of an Eye Patch

At the age of twenty-two I stood six foot four in my denim jacket, blue jeans and military shirt. I shared a small basement flat in Rathmines with Sebastian, a socialist who didn't believe in paying rent. I wanted to be a writer. I still wanted to play in a band. I wanted a girlfriend. I didn't know what I wanted.

I had seen The Clash at Trinity, an astonishingly noisy epic of a concert that seemed to be more about energy and attitude than music. I can still see the waves of spit from the audience raining down on Joe Strummer while he hung on the microphone stand as though he were having a psychotic episode. I remember guys boasting afterwards about having landed spits directly into Strummer's open gob.

I had overcome my heartbreak with Mary and had completed a degree in English and History. I got good marks (the highest I had achieved in my college career). The week after finishing I received a note from UCD's History Department. It went something like this:

Dear Mr Mac Anna

We are delighted that you have successfully completed your degree in History. However, no one in the department can recall ever having met you. It appears that you have completed your degree without ever having attended a tutorial. Do drop in to the department when you have a chance, if only to introduce yourself. We are all extremely curious.

There were few jobs going in Dublin. McClelland emigrated to Germany. Sherlock disappeared down the country. I bumped into a guy from my final year English class who told me he was heading for Zimbabwe. 'There are lots of opportunities there, now that things have settled down,' he said. 'You should think about it.'

So I thought about Zimbabwe. For about two and a half minutes.

Unbeknownst to me, my mother had put me down for jobs in the health service and the library. She filled out the application forms and sent them in. The first thing I knew about either was when I got a letter requiring me to attend a formal interview for a job as some kind of junior exec in the health service. I put on my one white shirt, a black tie and my best jacket and showed up at a hotel room in town. There were three old guys in suits and it all went along quite pleasantly until they asked me why I'd like a job in the health service.

'Because I need a job,' I told them.

They said they'd be in touch.

I didn't bother with the interview for the library job. Instead I decided to take an MA in Anglo-Irish Literature. I figured it would put off going into the world for a year at least – something was sure to come up.

I was summoned to the office of Professor McHugh, Professor of English at UCD, for an audience about my application to join the MA. If I passed this test, I wouldn't have to find a real job for a year or two at least. I wouldn't have to emi-grate to Zimbabwe. I could stay in college and remain young. That was, if I could convince Professor McHugh and his fel-lows that I was a worthy candidate for their course.

I was brought to a small, book-lined office where sat the august Professor McHugh, flanked by two other academics. All were dressed in tweed. They quizzed me for a while and asked me why I wanted to do an MA in Anglo-Irish Literature. I gave them some shite about Beckett and Joyce and my heritage, etc.

Professor McHugh squinted at me over his glasses. He want-ed to know what I intended to submit as my thesis. Off the top of my head, I said I wanted to write a novel while writing a the-sis about writing a novel. I wanted to combine the creative with the academic to present an original thesis. They were silent for a moment. Professor McHugh told me to leave it with them.

Afterwards, walking to the Belfield canteen, I felt that I had achieved a kind of victory. At least I hadn't gone for the nor-mal thing – a thesis on Joyce's influence on postmodernism and all that. On second thoughts maybe I'd blown it.

A week later I got a polite letter declining my idea for a the-sis but praising its originality. However, I was accepted for the MA in Anglo-Irish Literature. I could get back to them before Christmas with a new subject for my thesis.

They were being very decent about this.

It turned out that I was the only Irish person in a class com-posed of a couple dozen Americans and several Canadians. I found it hard to motivate myself to study – I kept feeling that I should be doing something else, something more worthwhile.

One morning an enthusiastic Canadian woman brought in a tape of Irish traditional music. 'It will get us in the right mood for reading Synge,' she explained. We listened to diddley-eye stuff for an hour. Afterwards everyone agreed that it had been a wonderful tutorial.

I considered switching to Icelandic studies – anything had to be better than that. I decided to skip all future tutorials.

Shortly after the diddley-eye tutorial, a professor called me aside. He wanted to know what I intended to submit as my thesis. I told him I wanted to write a novel while writing a thesis about writing a novel, to combine the creative with the academic.

He told me to leave it with him.

★

With summer coming, I figured I should get a part-time job. Somewhere away from Belfield.

One day I got a tip that there was a weekend job going selling punk badges on a stall in the Dandelion Market. The stall was run by a guy named John – I got his number and gave him a call.

John Fisher was taller than me. His friend and business partner, Eoin, seemed taller than him. My interview consisted of a discussion about the musical merits of The Sex Pistols.

I got the gig.

That Saturday morning, Grafton Street was sharp and cool and clear in vibrant sunshine. There was a Boomtown Rats poster on a hoarding.

We took trays of badges out of John's car and set up the stall in the middle of the Dandelion Market. On the way there we passed two middle-aged male buskers – the first was singing 'Blowing in the Wind' and the other was singing 'A Horse with No Name'.

A bunch of punks loitered outside Advance Records on King Street. They gave us the glare. A small guy in a frock coat with spiky blond hair stared at us with his hands on his hips, like he was thinking about leading a charge. I'd heard about this guy. His name was Reb and he was one of the very first punks in Dublin – and he took no prisoners.

We quickened our pace.

The whiff of hashish hit us as we got to the Dandelion

Market, which was like a filled-in bomb crater with stalls, many of which were located inside what appeared to be a huge aircraft hangar. There were leaks everywhere – it was always cold and permanently draughty. The smell of dope mingled with incense and Indian oil. There were some enclosed shops, but most of the trade consisted of hundreds of small stall holders, selling everything from carpets to hash pipes. Many of them looked they they'd just got back from Woodstock. Lots of hair. Lots of flares. Lots of woolly jumpers. There were some fabulous-looking girls.

While we were setting up, a girl with black curly hair bounced past. Our eyes met and she smiled. I reckoned I was going to like the Dandelion.

Our stall consisted of a large foldout table, upon which we set up ten hard cardboard trays of badges. Underneath we kept a small cashbox and two boxes containing extra badges in plastic bags.

Around eleven we were joined by Dave, a smiley bloke with a big nose. Dave and I ran the badges stall – John and Eoin dropped in to help out and take the money.

The Ramones and The Sex Pistols were big sellers, as were The Boomtown Rats, The Buzzcocks, The Damned, Blondie, X-Ray Spex, The Clash and The Snivelling Shits. The Snivelling Shits weren't really a band at all, John told me. 'They're just a bunch of eejits in Manchester having a lark.' But they were still popular.

Two beautiful brown-eyed girls bought a Boomtown Rats badge.

'Do you know Bob Geldof?' one of them asked me.

I told them that I knew him. (This was basically true. I had met him a few times and we knew each other by name. My ex-girlfriend's best friend had gone out with the Rats' bass player so I had spent a bit of time with the band and seen a few gigs. I had even attended the Rats' rehearsals in the front room of my ex-girlfriend's best friend's house. I felt that I knew Geldof as well as any other stall holder in the Dandelion.)

'I'd do anything to meet Bob Geldof,' she said, big brown eyes looking right into mine.

For a moment I couldn't speak. Instead I nodded. The girl continued staring. Her friend too. Four big, brown eyes drilled into me, seeking a reaction. I told them I'd see what I could do. Pleased, they went off.

It turned out that Dave played lead guitar. He had been in loads of bands and his last outfit – The Max Quod Band – had just broken up. The Max Quod Band had achieved notoriety in Dublin rock circles for firing their bass player, Adam Clayton. They told him that he couldn't play so he joined a new band – U2.

Not to be outdone, I told him that I was lead singer with Johnny Jurex and the Punk Pistols. Dave asked me how many gigs we'd played. 'A few,' I lied.

Dave liked the name Johnny Jurex. In those days getting the name right was crucial. Fit Kilkenny and the Remoulds had a good name. So too did Sacre Bleu, The Atrix, The Vipers, The Fabulous Fabrics and the magnificently monikered but never seen, Damian Leper and the Open Sores. A band named Free Booze always got enormous crowds to McGonagles.

Dave and I decided to form a band – or at least to form a name for a band.

We came up with Bing Crosby and the Golf Clubs. Too silly.

Then Elvis and the Necrophiliacs. Too obvious.

Finally, I suggested Eamon de Valera and the Gravediggers – it had promise and it was very punk and irreverent – but it still wasn't right.

We dropped the Eamon. Not punk enough.

Dave suggested Rocky and it fit – Rocky De Valera and the Gravediggers. It sounded great and was very punk.

So now we were a band. All we had to do was find a drummer and a bass player. Rehearsals, songs, gigs, records, that sort of stuff would be no problem. All that would happen once we got the right people in.

My confidence grew. It was a pleasant surprise that things were going so well. It usually took a long time to get the name right – and that was often the hardest bit. Nobody wanted to be lumbered with a crap name. Just ask The Bunko Squad or The Great Saturday Night Swindle.

We made plans. Discussed songs we wanted to cover. Songs by Dr Feelgood, The Ramones, The Pirates, Robert Gordon. 'Brand New Cadillac' by Vince Taylor and the Playboys, a fifties rock-and-roll cult classic. No boring old stuff. Dave was a big fan of The Jam, but we eventually decided against doing any punk covers. We didn't want to be like the punks who knocked around outside Advance. We wanted to have our own identity. We wanted to be a new, modern, no-nonsense rock-and-roll band. A band with the attitude and energy of punk. A band as exciting as Dr Feelgood or The Pirates or even The Stranglers, who were really good musicians.

I loved the fact that I was in a band. No more boring MA and I wouldn't have to emigrate to Zimbabwe.

At lunchtime I strolled past the bouncy girl and gave her a big smile. Bouncy smiled back. I rambled down Grafton Street, passing the Boomtown Rats poster and the bloke who was still singing, 'I've been through the desert on a horse with no name.'

I was in a band and the name was Rocky. Rocky De Valera.

★

A shed in Howth.

We were in someone's shed in Howth.

Dave set up his guitar and amplifier. Rob, an economics student from Howth, sat behind his drum kit while Sgt Floyd Pepper from The Muppets (Tony, another student) plugged his bass guitar into a small amp. Rob had brought a rhythm guitarist, his friend Nicky – tall, tough looking, didn't say much.

The shed was dark and dank and smelled like it had been used for gutting fish. Rob had borrowed it for the day, the deal being that we cleaned up after ourselves.

We hit a problem – there were no microphones. In my haste to arrange the rehearsal, I had forgotten to organise a mike for myself, the lead singer. In the end I had to settle for a broom handle.

We launched into 'Brand New Cadillac'. The guitars sounded louder than a jet engine. I started to sing into the broom handle. I couldn't hear a thing, and neither could anyone else – but it felt great.

Paul Brown watched us intently from the side of the room. A big man, Paul was already something of a Howth legend – he'd played with a number of bands, including Rat Salad, and was regarded as a genius of the bass guitar. He was ostensibly there to make sure we didn't destroy the shed.

Even at that early stage it was obvious to everyone that Dave was a gifted guitarist. Nobody was taking much notice of me (maybe because in the world of musicians, ability is crucial). They couldn't hear me anyway and so couldn't tell if I was any good or not.

I decided that I shouldn't let not having a proper microphone get in the way of my performance. So I danced around, trying some of the shapes thrown by the singer from The Radiators. Then I tried out the Jim Morrison lurch – leaning into the mike stand and allowing it to slip, so that you lurched across the stage like a drunk.

Soon everyone was watching me. I made them laugh, but I also reminded them that I was in the shed too.

We played some Dr Feelgood numbers, then 'Chantilly Lace' by the Big Bopper. We did 'Don't Munchen It' by The Pirates, 'Midnight Shift' by Buddy Holly, 'Lucille' by Little

Richard and a Robert Gordon number, 'Red Hot'. Every song was played superfast with maximum energy – in other words, punked up. We didn't play anything by The Ramones or The Sex Pistols. We were a rock band with a punk attitude; that's how we saw it anyway.

We rehearsed for two hours. At the end we were tired and sweating. I felt exhausted but exhilarated. This was what I wanted to do. This was fate calling, showing me the road to take for the rest of my life. I wanted to play a gig immediately.

'What do you think?' I asked them.

'Sounds good,' Dave said. 'We've definitely got something.'

'Are we a band?' I asked.

'Yeah,' Dave said. The others nodded. Big Paul Brown shrugged.

'Good,' I said. 'Because we've got a gig next Tuesday.'

On the morning of our first gig I got up at seven and spent an hour getting ready. Mostly, though, I walked about the flat poking at things, which drove Sebastian the Socialist mad. I hated our apartment, but it was cheap.

Sebastian the Socialist occupied the main room because he got there first. I inhabited the 'cave', a tiny room behind the kitchen where there was scarcely room for a bed and where I couldn't stand up. Unless you entered the room at a crouch, you whacked your skull off the low-curved ceiling. Once I brought a girl back to my cave and she took one look and walked out. 'How can anyone live in such squalor?' she said.

A quiet guy in his late twenties named Desmond lived in the room behind us. Desmond liked to play the blues and sometimes in the evenings we heard him singing 'Crossroads', twanging away on a nylon-stringed guitar.

Occasionally, Desmond's friend Winston the Poet stayed with him. Winston had done Primal Scream Therapy. Then he started writing Primal Scream Poetry. Sometimes we heard him screaming out his Primal Scream Verses.

The weekend I moved in, a junkie stole my entire record collection. Ten Years After, The Doors, Atomic Rooster, Joni Mitchell, Allman Bros, Little Feat – all gone. Since then I'd managed to buy new albums, including The Ramones, The Stranglers, Blondie and Robert Gordon, along with The Saints and some punk as well as old rock-and-roll singles. Sometimes when I went out at night I stuck my records under my mattress, resulting in several becoming warped and unplayable.

I told myself that the burglary helped me to shed the old and get into the new, but that's not much compensation for losing your life's collection of albums. The truth was that I was dying to get out of the flat and move someplace decent, but I couldn't afford it. I was stuck living in the kip.

I put on jeans and a white shirt and my imitation leather jacket (plastic) that I bought for fifteen pounds in a shop on Capel Street. To finish off the look, I ran some silver chains I'd found in a skip through the lapels of my jacket, connecting them to the buttonholes in the flaps over the pockets. 'Very scary,' Sebastian the Socialist said. 'You look like a student in a plastic jacket.' Then he turned over and went back to sleep.

I studied my image in the mirror. He was right. My image was lacking. I needed something else, something edgy and attention grabbing.

I flicked through my album collection for inspiration and found a cover shot of Johnny Kidd and the Pirates – Johnny was wearing a black eye patch and looked cool and menacing. Just the thing.

I hurried from the basement flat and walked to the local chemist in Rathmines, where they offered me a white eye patch. 'No, it has to be black,' I told them. They didn't have one so I walked to another chemist. Same story. Then I tried another.

Eventually I found a chemist that had black eye patches. I tried one on. It looked very menacing. I couldn't see a thing on my left side, but so what? I'd be careful.

To test it out I wore the eye patch on the way home. Some people stepped out of my way, or so I imagined.

★

Our first gig was in the Belfield bar at lunchtime. It was a real gig and not a doss like Johnny Jurex. We had had three rehearsals – though, as yet, I still hadn't managed to sing into a microphone and had no idea what my singing voice sounded like, or if I could even sing. Nevertheless, I was confident.

A week earlier we had recruited a sixth member, Baz, a saxophonist. X-Ray Spex had a sax player. Now we had Baz.

It felt like my birthday, I was so excited. I was the singer in a six-piece, punk-rock, new-wave, rock-and-roll band. I knew we were ready.

At ten when we arrived at the bar, it was empty except for the bar staff and a large PA system. We started setting up. By eleven fifteen, we had had our first sound check and I finally sang into a real microphone. The power and clamour was immense. I thought we sounded magnificent.

Afterwards, Baz was encouraging. 'Your voice doesn't do that melody thing yet. But that will come in time. The important thing is to keep singing.'

'Huh?'

I had no idea what he was on about.

I kept the eye patch on for a while, just in case anyone wandered in. Then I decided that it should be a surprise so I put it into a small cigarette packet and into my pocket. My secret weapon.

We drank a round of pints to get us warmed up and to calm our nerves. Then we ordered another round. I kept busy so that I wouldn't have to think about how anxious I was. Keeping busy meant constantly dashing to the bathroom to adjust my chains in the mirror.

Before the gig, we posed in our dressing room – the pub toilets – so that a speccy first-year guy we knew could take a photo of us. Our first photo session.

Then somebody announced us and we went out onto the stage. The place was packed. We started with 'Peter Gun', then went into 'Shakin' All Over'. It was like a riot. At some stage I threw myself into the front rows and the front rows threw me back. The crowd loved us and we got three encores.

Afterwards we sat in the bar, drenched in sweat but beaming with satisfaction. People came up to congratulate us. We were bought pints. A Students' Union guy came up and booked us for a lunchtime open-air gig the following week. I decided that I would not be completing my Master's after all. There would be no more lectures. No more tutorials. No thesis. I was enrolled full-time in the University of Rock.

We were a gigging band. We had arrived.

Later, intoxicated with the morning's work, I met my friend Pat, who I used to play pool with. It was nearly four in the afternoon and he wanted to go for breakfast.

Pat was tall and robust and looked like a young Kris Kristofferson. He had an immense effect on women – he was the charming bad guy they wanted to tame. He once came with me to dinner with a girl I fancied and ended up going off with the girl himself. The next morning he called round to apologise. I didn't hold a grudge, we were good friends – I just didn't introduce him to girls I liked. Pat was either repeating second year or had just finished his third. He may have dropped out altogether. Nobody knew and Pat didn't seem too bothered about his situation.

He saw the gig and thought we were terrific. He said all we needed was to find a good manager and then we could go all the way.

We walked to Rathmines to get food, but neither of us had any money. We stopped outside the supermarket. 'Hang on here a second,' Pat said. 'I'll make a few enquiries.'

I waited outside in my leather jacket. After a few minutes I took off the eye patch and put it in my pocket. Best to keep it for stage wear, I decided, otherwise I might really go blind. After three hours behind the patch, my eye felt weird, like it had been smudged by a giant thumb.

Pat came out. He opened his jacket to reveal a packet of rashers and a box of eggs. 'I'm just borrowing these,' he said. 'I'll drop the money in later when I get some.'

We went back to my apartment and cooked up breakfast only to discover that we didn't have any coffee. 'Don't worry,' Pat said. He went out and came back twenty minutes later with a jar of instant. 'I made the same arrangements.'

I spent the rest of the day in a delightful daze. I felt as though I had arrived at the beginning of my life's work. I would write and sing brilliant songs. I would tour the world with the band. I would never have to take a nine to five. I wouldn't have to write a thesis that combined the creative with the academic.

'Keep me in mind when you're looking for a manager,' Pat said.

That night we went to a party in the apartment upstairs, which was occupied by Ron and Stan, two chaps who ran Snotz, Dublin's first mobile punk disco.

The room was packed with students, punks, a few hippies and several off-duty accountants.

The party went well until Stan put on a non-punk single, 'Tin Man' by America. Ron saw this as a betrayal of the principles of Snotz. The disco was all about playing punk and new wave, it was set up in opposition to bland dinosaurs like America. Stan didn't see it that way anymore. 'I am not going to allow my personal tastes to be held back by the imperialism of punk,' he said.

After that, the party fizzled out.

★

At ten in the morning, the steps outside the Administration Building in UCD were deserted.

The day was sharp, with a cold breeze. There were few students around. The Students' Union had booked us to play a lunchtime gig to launch the new campaign against high fees. The union would pay for the PA and equipment, all we had to do was to order the amps from the Band Centre. We would just show up and play. It would cost us nothing and would be a great way for the band to pick up some momentum – and some free publicity.

I went into the Arts Building and found a pay phone. I called the Band Centre and ordered the amps for the gig. 'The amps must be delivered before noon,' I specified.

'No problem,' Band Centre Guy said. 'Now what's the name of the band?'

'Rocky De Valera and the Gravediggers.'

There was a moment between us on the phone. 'Is this some kind of a fucking joke?' Band Centre Guy said. 'Are you taking the piss?'

I was shocked. I assured Band Centre Guy that we were a real band, that his amps would be paid for and that this was not a Rag Week wind-up. Finally he relented and agreed to deliver the gear before noon.

I went back to the Admin steps and waited around for half an hour, feeling a bit of a tool – not an auspicious start to the second gig of a rock-and-roll career. The singer should not have to wait around for the rest of the band. Not very professional.

Then Dave arrived with a big grin on his face, carrying his guitar. I was reassured. I was convinced Dave was the best guitarist in Ireland. He was as good as Wilko Johnston from Dr Feelgood and better than all the punk players, but then that wouldn't be hard, as the punks would probably have admitted.

Soon, Rob and Nicky pulled up in a car. We carried Rob's

drums onto the steps and helped him set up. Finally Tony shuf-
fled towards us, toting his bass on his back.

Our self-appointed roadie, Rocker, turned up. Rocker was a
quiet-spoken, unflappable Englishman who wore a real leather
jacket. For a while in England he had been a biker, though he
admitted that he had belonged to a very polite gang who lived
for motorbikes and bike rallies and never got into any trouble.
Nevertheless, in our eyes Rocker was the real thing. We ignored
the tin whistle that he kept in his inside pocket, along with a
Teach Yourself Book of Irish Jigs.

By eleven thirty, there was still no sign of the PA system or
the hired amplifiers, so we stood around on the steps, in our
leather jackets, trying to look as though we knew what was
going on. The guy from the Students' Union said that Band
Centre Guy was on his way.

By twelve fifteen, there was still no PA. We were frozen and
confused.

Did this mean the gig was cancelled? We consulted the
Students' Union guy. 'No way,' he said. 'The PA will be here.
Sure, don't we have to make speeches?'

At twelve twenty-five, a large van pulled up in front of the
steps and a guy got out. 'Is this where the gig is happening?' he
asked and we nodded.

The guy from the Band Centre began to haul gear out of the
back of his van and, by twelve forty-five, all the amplifiers were
working and the mike stands were in place – but there were no
working microphones because Band Centre Guy hadn't yet
finished setting up the sound desk.

So we had to wait.

Some students showed up. The guy from the Students'
Union wanted us to play for forty minutes. '*The Irish Times* is
coming,' he explained. They were hoping for big coverage for
the start of the fees campaign. Our job was to draw a big crowd
for the speeches. Someone had forgotten to distribute posters,

but the guy assured us that word of mouth would bring the students out. Afterwards, the pints were on the union.

Eventually, the mikes were working. We did a quick sound check – we played 'Lucille' by Little Richard, one of rock music's first punks. I heard my voice coming back to me through the on-stage monitors and was surprised at the power and the punch. It was so different to be playing out in the open instead of inside a stuffy bar room. I loved the way the sound seemed to bounce back from the library walls. I could feel my voice gliding across the lake, stopping people in their tracks. Cars slowed down. People on bicycles changed direction to check us out.

My voice definitely did have that 'melodic thing'; it sounded grand to me. I didn't know what Baz was talking about. Besides, how melodic did a voice have to be to sing 'Shakin' All Over'?

A crowd of students appeared, drawn by the sound check. The day suddenly brightened.

We huddled together at the side of the stage to work out a big entrance. We couldn't just walk on and start playing – there had to be some drama. We decided that the band would start with an instrumental, 'Peter Gunn'. After a few minutes, I would roar on stage on the back of Rocker's motorbike, jump off the bike and, at my signal, the band would go into 'Shakin' All Over'.

Very rock and roll.

One fifteen. Time to get ready. The band tuned up and Rocker and I made our way to the motorbike. We had gone about five paces when we were hailed by a delegation of students. Four small, young women approached, all wearing glasses and serious faces. Their leader came straight to the point. They were not happy with the sexist nature of the band's songs. They wanted us to change the line 'Lucille, you don't do your daddy's will.' The line could be misconstrued and they

Mr Cravat and Mr Earring

Fergus Bourke took this photograph of my father and me for *The Sunday Tribune*'s 'Kindred' series in 1984. Dad was still into cravats and I still wore an earring.

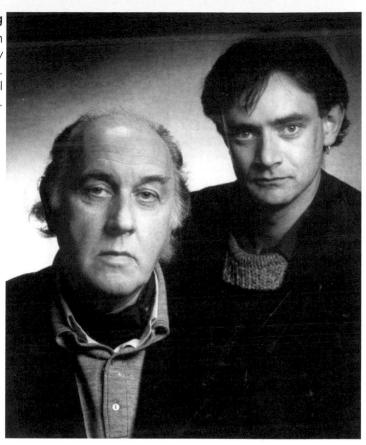

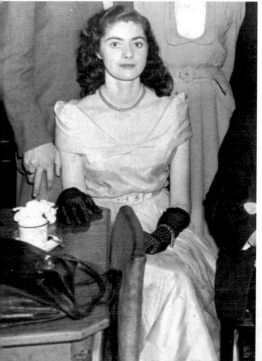

My mother at the Guild Actors Equity Ball in 1952

This was taken before my mother met my dad, she was already renowned for her good looks and auburn hair.

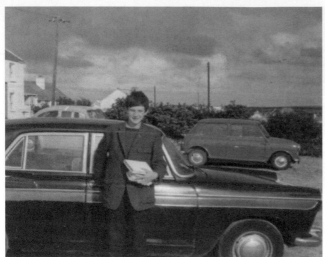

Ferdia's first tour

Dad took this photo of me standing beside his Austin Cambridge. We were in Donegal where Dad was adjudicating at a drama festival. I had brought along a supply of Kurt Vonneguts and Ray Bradburys.

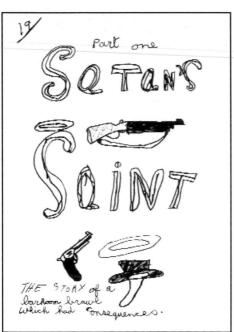

Fifth Class devil

My story about a gungslinger who was possessed by the devil caused hell within our Authors' Club of eleven-year-olds.

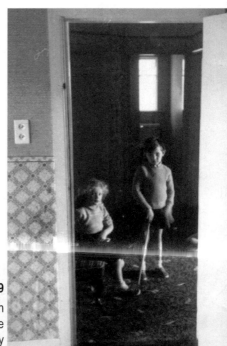

Killiney, 1959

My sister and me in the 'house with no furniture' in Killiney – sometime after attempting to assassinate my mother with a three-prong plug.

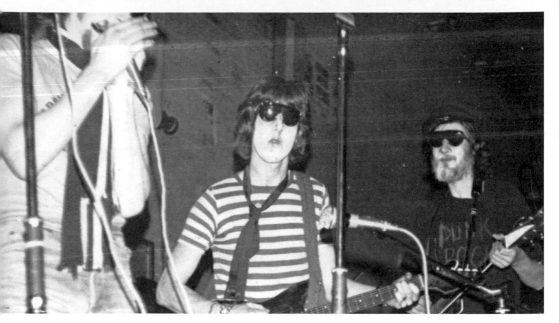

Anarchy in Belfield

Johnny Jurex and the Punk Pistols rock Theatre L in Belfield Rag Week, 1976
From left: Charlie Jurex (harmonica), Jimi Jurex (Seamus McClelland) and Johnny Jurex (me). Moments after this photo was snapped someone sprayed the stage with a fire hose and nearly fried us all.

The human light bulb and Mary
Eamon 'Sherlock' Holmes experiences a light bulb moment as drummer with Johnny Jurex. Note the unusual human cymbal stand. Also in the photo is Mary from Cork, strumming away on her two-string guitar. I was too shy to ask her out but had no problem asking her to join a punk 'doss' band.

Back to mono

Rocky De Valera and the Gravediggers strike an elegant pose backstage in McGonagles in early 1978. The eye patch is made from a shade from a broken pair of sunglasses with a Celtic cross stuck on with super glue. My leather jacket is real but the chains are all plastic. The legendary Jack Dublin is on the left holding my leash. *From left*: Jack (bass), me, Harpo (drums), Pierre Parnell (rhythm guitar) and Dave Hero (guitar).

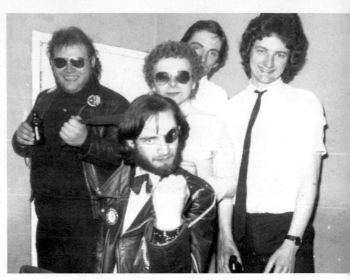

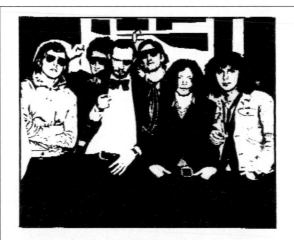

Our first photo shoot and poster, Dublin 1978

The very first line-up of Rocky De Valera and the Gravediggers pose in the toilets of the Belfield Bar before our lunchtime debut. The dicky bow seemed like a good idea at the time. Baz, the saxophonist (our answer to X-Ray Spex), is on the extreme right.

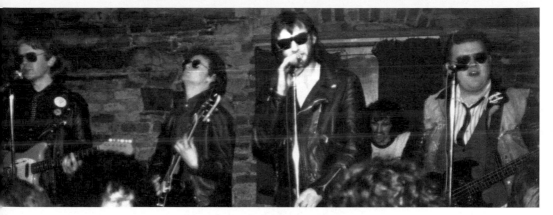

Big Bad Biker Band play Toners

This photograph accompanied a good review by Ian Wilson for *In Dublin* magazine in 1979. The drummer is Dave 'Bucko' Buckley.

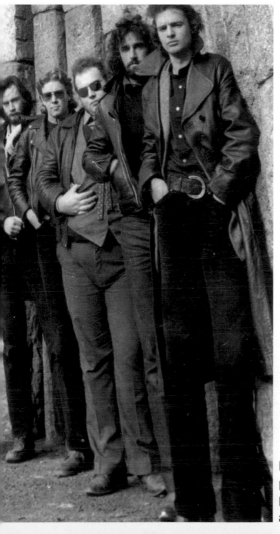

Rock and Roll makes you taller

Even The Lizard is taller than me in this photo. Rocky De Valera and the Gravediggers perfect our acclaimed alleyway pose in Dublin in 1978.

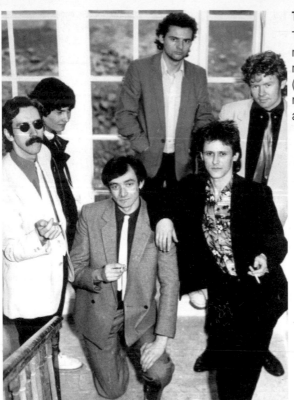

This band is jinxed

The Rhythm Kings experience a Simple Minds moment. This photo was taken on the stairway of my apartment in Mountjoy Square in 1981. Clint (*extreme left*) is the only one who looks like a rock 'n' roller, the rest of us look like defrocked advertising executives.

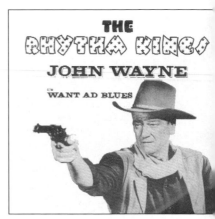

Is it yer man?

'John Wayne' reached number twenty-seven in the Irish Top Thirty before dropping out of the charts because we ran out of copies. The song, which was written in five minutes, became our mad ska anthem: 'Is it a bird, is it a plane, no, no – it's John Wayne.' Don't know why it didn't catch on worldwide.

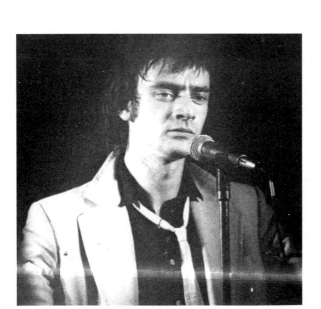

Why Figi?

My reaction upon receiving the news that The Rhythm Kings had been offered a two-day tour of Fiji. After some deliberation we declined the invitation, along with a later offer of a one-day tour of East Berlin.

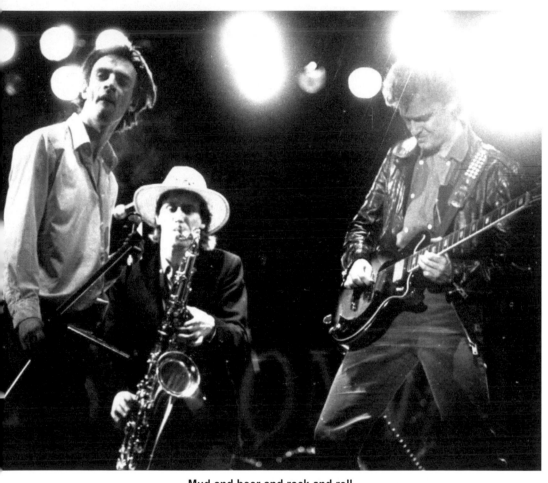

Mud and beer and rock and roll

Playing live was always the best part. The Rhythm Kings gigged all over Ireland but reserved something special for the big summer festivals – this was taken at Lisdoonvarna in 1981.
(*From left*: Rocky, The Individual, The Lizard)

Horror movies kept me safe

After cancer, I carried on wearing my beret indoors for a long time, even after my hair grew back. This photo was taken in our apartment in Dalkey in 1988. I had surrounded myself with books and posters from B-movies like *Basket Case* and *Night of the Living Dead*. For some reason, the horror posters made me feel safe.

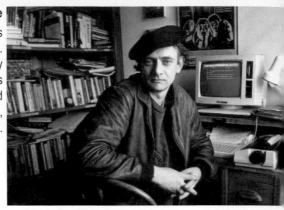

People's Park, Dún Laoghaire, 1991

One day Kate started taking measurements of my head, before disappearing into the back room. I thought she was going to have me committed, instead she was making fez-type hats to keep my bald head warm. This hat is my favourite and I still have it.

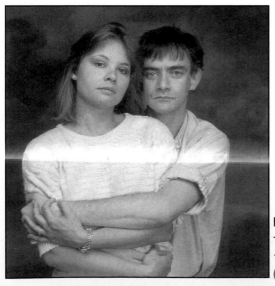

Before the storm

This photo of an optimistic young couple was taken in 1984, shortly after we were married in Cape Cod (following a three-month courtship).

didn't want the Students' Union to be a party to that type of blatant sexism.

A discussion ensued in which I told them that I didn't write the song. It was written in the fifties by Little Richard.

'That's no concern of ours,' the delegation leader stated. 'The line must be changed or the show doesn't go ahead.'

I protested, but after a while I could see that this delegation was unmoved. I gave up arguing. It was pointless and, besides, I wanted to play this gig. 'OK, I'll sing something else,' I promised.

'Oh, one more thing,' smiled the leader. 'We would appreciate it if you didn't use the word "baby" in any of the songs – it's demeaning to women.'

Rocker's motorbike turned out to be a Yamaha 50, one of the smallest bikes on the road. I climbed on and stuck up like a flagpole. I began to think that arriving on stage on the back of a Yamaha 50 might not be as spectacular an opening as we had thought.

The band went into 'Peter Gunn'. Rocker started the bike. We drove through a large crowd of students onto the side of the steps. I leapt off and dashed up the remaining steps to the makeshift stage. With the eye patch on my vision was impaired, and in my haste I smacked myself in my good eye with the microphone. Now I couldn't see anything. The band charged into 'Shakin' All Over'. I started singing. I remained totally blind for the first two verses.

The sound was rough. My voice sounded as though it was being relayed a few seconds late through the cacophony of an erupting volcano. We played six or seven songs. We did 'Lucille', but I forgot to alter the words. It was all I could do to remember any of the words to the songs, let alone change them. The young, bespectacled women approached the stage and started shouting at me, but I couldn't hear them over the music.

Halfway through 'Brand New Cadillac', the Students' Union guy came up to us with a megaphone and told us to stop. Our second gig was over. The crowd gave us some polite applause. Some people were laughing. Most seemed to be wearing big grins on their faces.

We packed up our gear and went to the bar. We could hear speeches beginning behind us. The crowd thinned rapidly – nothing clears a space more quickly than student politics.

In the bar, we drank pints and relaxed. The buzz inside my head made me feel invincible, like a superhero. I had never felt this good about myself or the world. I may not have discovered the meaning of life, but at least I had found the meaning of *my* life.

That night I accompanied Sebastian the Socialist to a left-wing party in a big Georgian house up the road. The place was packed with hippies and radicals and various denim-clad lefties. I wore my old denim jacket that I'd covered with badges from the stall in the Dandelion Market. By covering it in badges I hoped that nobody would notice that I was wearing denim, the uniform of the oppressive hippy music dictatorship. I also hoped that John and Eoin didn't find out that I had borrowed about five hundred of their badges.

At the party, some people were impressed by my jacket of badges. One man came up to me to study the badges. He fingered a Ramones badge on my lapel. 'Oh, I see you like Ramon-eesh,' he exclaimed. 'I've read all his pamphlets on the migration of the working classes. The man's a genius.'

Another man came up to ask me what party I represented. I told him that I sold rock badges from a stall in the Dandelion Market. 'You're a commercial vendor,' he fumed. 'I thought you were serious.'

He then went to leave the room. Even though both his hands were free, he kicked the door and continued kicking it until someone on the other side opened it. Then he went through, waving his hands in outrage. 'That's Gerald,' Sebastian the Socialist explained. 'He doesn't believe in doorknobs.'

Pat called over the next morning with *The Irish Times*. Rocky De Valera and the Gravediggers had made it onto the front page. The band was mentioned in the report on UCD Students' Union's mass rally on campus to protest against a hike in college fees. I scanned the paper and read and re-read our band name. It appeared as though we were being guided by destiny. You didn't get the name of your band on the front page of *The Irish Times* unless you were going places. Even Sebastian the Socialist was impressed.

I gave up going into college altogether. There was no point. I was going to make it as a rock star.

That night I met Jane, a girl I'd been seeing for a few weeks, and told her that I may not be around for much longer. 'Why not?' she asked.

I told her that I would probably have made it big by Christmas. She laughed so hard that I thought she was choking on something. 'Are you OK? Was it something I said?'

12

The Name is De Valera,
Rocky De Valera

We met at nine every morning in my flat in Rathmines, which became the rehearsal space. Sebastian the Socialist slept through most of our rehearsals, even though the drums were next to his head.

One night Desmond and Winston came over and we bought beer and wine. Pat arrived, followed by Rocker. We instigated a boozy jam session. Desmond played the blues and I messed about with my old, battered two-string guitar and attempted to play slide with a beer bottle. The drunker we got, the better it sounded.

At some stage, someone put on Rocker's motorbike helmet and invited me to smash the battered guitar on it. I whacked the helmet with the guitar. Suddenly it seemed like a brilliant idea. We took turns putting on Rocker's helmet while someone else whacked it with the old two-string guitar. I wondered if we could use this stunt on stage, though people would probably just think that we were copying The Who. Everyone fell about laughing except Winston, who thought that this was a sacrilege against music. Winston tried Primal Screaming us into quitting, but Eddie and the Hot Rods were singing 'Get Out of Denver' on the stereo and the rest of us were laughing and whacking each other on the helmet so nobody paid any heed to him. The music finished at the same instant that the old guitar fell to pieces.

Winston's face turned red and he yelled, 'Don't you people realise what you have done? You have destroyed an instrument that God intended to make music. You had no right to do that. You should have given it to someone who has a need for it.'

I explained that the guitar was old and battered and had cracks and holes in it and was no good for anything. Besides, it was mine. I could do what I wanted with my own guitar.

Pat stepped in to have his say. 'This thing is not about a guitar. It's about freedom of expression.'

Suddenly Desmond became enraged. 'Since when is wanton destruction a freedom of expression?'

Pat wanted to know why Desmond was so upset. After all, he'd taken part in the destruction or maybe he was just following orders. Desmond went ballistic. 'We're talking about blasphemy here,' he yelled.

A spot of pushing broke out and the row shifted direction. Now it was about hospitality. No one had the right to criticise another person for their behaviour in their own place, especially if that behaviour was not hurting anyone. Next the argument switched to punk lyrics versus real poetry. 'Bob Dylan is the only real poet,' Desmond shouted. 'Dylan and Robert Johnson. You can stuff your Johnny Rottens up your arses.'

Pat tried to calm everyone down. I lost track of the reason everyone was shouting. The argument started off about the guitar, had progressed rapidly to the demerits of punk and now it was about shouting for its own sake. Everyone was too out of it to stop. Eventually things calmed down and we sat around in the apartment, leaving the broken bits of guitar where they were.

Winston said that the row would never have happened if we hadn't wrecked a sacred instrument. 'A guitar is a beautiful woman,' he said, eyes cloudy with tears. 'Why do you want to smash up a beautiful woman?' Nobody had an answer to that.

★

One day in the Dandelion Market a couple of weeks after the UCD gig, the singer from Fit Kilkenny and the Remoulds approached me at the badges stall. Fit Kilkenny and the Remoulds couldn't do their regular Thursday night gig at the Magnet in Pearse Street. Would Rocky De Valera and the Gravediggers be interested in standing in for two weeks?

Abso-fucking-lutely.

We got posters printed and covered the town. We bought Sellotape and stuck the posters to poles and walls and post-boxes. When we returned later on, we were amazed to find the posters gone. So we stuck up new posters. This time we Sellotaped our posters over existing posters of bands like Sacre Bleu, The Resistors, Revolver and DC Nien.

Rocker designed Rocky De Valera and the Gravediggers badges. We got them pressed and printed in a shop called Crazy Horse Corner and then swanned about proudly in the Dandelion Market and on Grafton Street, sporting our new Gravediggers identities, though we were careful not to hang around for too long outside Advance Records on King Street – we didn't want to get sneered at by the punks or risk getting into a fight.

Advance Records was an intimidating place to buy a record, but it was the only record shop in town that stocked all the latest punk and new-wave releases, including those on Stiff, Chiswick and other English labels.

The punks sneered at hippies and others who passed. They saved a lot of their venom for bands, especially Dublin new-wave bands such as The Atrix or U2. They give U2 a particularly robust slagging whenever they passed by because U2 seemed sincere and were polite to everyone and the Grafton Street punks hated that.

Rocker and I hit the Berni Inn for a drink. We were sipping pints at a table in the back room when the band Revolver came in. Revolver had released a single, 'Silently Screaming', that had been favourably reviewed in the British music press. The band and its entourage took over a couple of tables and ordered drinks. I noticed that there were several gorgeous blonde girls with the band. The prettiest sat on Phil, the bass player's, knees – he looked like a young Greek god. At that moment it seemed to me that those bastards were living the life that I wanted to live. That realisation only made me more impatient. I told Rocker to hurry up, we'd got to move.

'Where to?' he asked.

'Anywhere,' I said, 'as long as we're moving.'

In the Dandelion, I flirted with Bouncy and told her I was in a band. I told her the name and showed her my badge and she was impressed. I asked her out and she said OK.

Later that week, we went on dates. One night Bouncy came back to my cave – she didn't think it was too bad, she found the low, curved ceiling 'funny'.

At weekends, my brother Niall hung around with us. He wore a real leather jacket. Whenever Niall, Rocker, Dave and myself, as well as several others, got together to walk down Grafton Street or around Rathmines, we looked like a biker gang in our black jackets.

In the flat we threw a big party to celebrate our impending first gig in the real world. We put on Robert Gordon and danced around the place. Niall revealed a real prowess for dancing, his long legs going like Spider-man. We all wanted to dance like him, but none of us was up to it.

★

The Magnet bar smelled of sweat and stale booze. We went through a vigorous sound check like proper professionals and then worked out a new stage act. We needed to mess with people's heads a bit more, I said. I decided that the Gravediggers should carry me on stage and prop me up against a microphone stand. At the first power chord, I would resurrect like the king of the zombies.

On the night, two guys from *Hot Press* arrived and sat at a front-row table. Backstage someone said that every band in town was in the audience, including the mysterious Damian Leper from the much-talked-about-but-never-seen-except-on-posters-and-wall-graffiti Damian Leper and the Open Sores.

We tried our big new opening. The band carried me out, propped me against the microphone stand and went back to get their guitars – I heard their footsteps retreating and the giggles of people in the audience and suddenly I felt very alone. What if they didn't come back?

The band seemed to be gone a long time and the audience began to shift in their chairs. I heard coughs and sighs and an occasional laugh. There were no catcalls and no slagging. People were genuinely intrigued.

Finally the Gravediggers returned. Dave struck a power chord. I sprang up suddenly, glaring into the audience out of my good eye. Instead of a loud, fast number we went into 'Pledging my Love', an old soulful song by the fifties cult hero Johnny Ace.

Some of the audience were intrigued, others were gobsmacked. I noticed that the two guys from *Hot Press* were falling about laughing. Why were the fuckers laughing? What was so funny about my singing?

We swung into 'Red Hot'. The two guys from *Hot Press* cracked up completely.

To stop them laughing I leapt onto their table, but the table collapsed, spilling drinks and beer mats everywhere. Everyone in the room cracked up.

Somehow, I regained my balance and the gig continued. My performance grew even wilder. I threw myself into the audience, only to fall down and accidentally tip a pint over my groin. I hurt my knee. I ripped open my shirt dramatically, shooting the buttons into the audience. A button plopped in some girl's vodka.

We got three encores. At the end of the night I invited the audience back to Rathmines for a big party.

Afterwards, everyone said it had been a fantastic gig. The two guys from *Hot Press* had disappeared. We figured that they must be going to review us. Pat wanted to know why the fuckers were laughing. 'I was thinking I might have to take them out,' he said quietly.

Someone introduced me to Damian Leper – a quiet, thoughtful nerd with thick glasses in a white nylon shirt. He promised that his band would be gigging before the end of the month. He had enjoyed our gig, but his band was better. I told him that I was looking forward to seeing the Open Sores. We shook hands and wished each other well before he disappeared into the night.

That was the last that I ever saw or heard of Damian Leper and the Open Sores, though their graffiti remained around town for many months.

Afterwards, the basement flat in Rathmines was crowded. It seemed as though the entire Magnet audience had turned up.

Just when the party was at its loudest and wildest, a bottle crashed through the window. We all rushed out but whoever threw it had scarpered. Angry and feeling violated on our big night, we tidied away the broken glass and taped a Ramones album cover over the hole in the window – then we got on with the party.

A little later, someone outside gave the door an enormous thump. I grabbed a broken chair leg and threw open the door ready to crown the bastard who had broken our window. The two *Hot Press* guys threw up their hands. 'Don't hit us, we're from *Hot Press*.'

It was a while before we believed their story, that they just wanted to come in to the party. When the excitement died down, Pat sidled up to me. 'You know those two guys from *Hot Press*?'

I glanced over at the record player where the they had taken over and were putting on a Rolling Stones record.

'Yes,' I said. 'What about them?'

Pat stared across the room at them meaningfully, 'You should have whacked them with the chair leg.'

★

I insisted to everyone that we were a professional rock band and that we must all be ready to sign a record deal and leave the country to tour the US or England at short notice. Some of the others didn't want to go professional. Baz left. So did the drummer. So we got a new drummer and rhythm guitarist. The bassist went back to his studies, so Paul from Howth joined. I gave Paul the stage name of Jack Dublin. He had no objections. Everyone needed to have a stage name. All of a sudden Dave Hero and I were the only originals left.

We played another Magnet gig that also went well. We were veterans of the rock world. I couldn't understand why the record companies weren't rushing to sign us up. Had they not heard about the effect our music and performances had on audiences?

I became deluded. I wanted the band to be travelling at the same fast rate of knots as my speeding brain. I drove the others mad by insisting on rehearsals at nine every morning and black leather jackets for everyone.

That night in Slattery's a guy came over to talk to us. He wanted to know the name of my favourite singer. I was still at the peak of my deluded phase. 'Rocky De Valera,' I told him.

The guy laughed. 'No seriously, now, what do you think of Geldof? Do you think he's a good singer?'

'Sure,' I said. 'Only he's not as good as me.'

The guy snapped and called me an 'ego-tripping fuckhead' and the 'cockiest loudmouth' he'd ever met in his life.

'I was just telling the truth,' I said casually and the guy's eyes completely popped. He made a lunge at me but Pat stepped between us. 'If you don't want to know the answers, don't ask questions,' Pat told the guy.

During rehearsal the next morning, I had trouble singing 'Sea Cruise', an old Frankie Ford song that we were trying to learn. 'That song's probably in the wrong key for you,' Dave said.

Wrong key? What was he talking about?

Dave explained that a song or piece of music was always in a certain key. If that key didn't suit a singer's voice, then it was possible to change the key. So we messed about with various keys. It turned out that the key of A suited my voice on that particular song.

I announced that from now on I wanted all songs to be in the key of A. The others rolled their eyes to heaven.

★

One afternoon I bumped into Reb outside Advance Records on King Street. Reb was still small, blond and belligerent. I had never seen him smile, he looked like a miniature Johnny Rotten and was always scowling at people – all bristle and attitude.

Now Reb blocked the doorway of Advance Records, arms folded. He stood five foot nothing and wore a long black coat and a chain but didn't have any safety pins.

I towered over him but he scared the shit out of me.

'What do you want?' he asked.

I blurted that I was thinking of buying the new one by The Damned. Reb shook his head. 'No,' he said. 'What's it all about?'

I didn't know what to say.

'It's about music, it's not about posing,' Reb explained.

'Right,' I said.

Reb fired off a few more questions, spat out of the side of his mouth like bullets. I was aware that if I failed this test, I would be fair game for all the other punks outside Advance Records.

After a while, Reb shrugged. I must have passed his street-credibility exam.

We began a proper conversation and he turned out to be OK. You didn't have to be a punk to impress him. He hated poseurs. Posing was the big crime. He hated the weekend punks and all the wannabe new wavers and all the fashion victims in their jumpers with the tailor-made holes in them.

He asked me about my influences and I told him that I liked The Ramones and Dr Feelgood as well as old rock and rollers like Charlie Feathers and Sonny Burgess.

He decided that I was OK – for the moment. 'Good luck with the band,' he said. 'I might come and see you some time.'

★

We embarked on a mini-tour of Kerry and Cork, so we hired a van driver and van, plus amplifiers and PA system.

Our first gig, in the Abbey Inn in Tralee, coincided with a local Fianna Fáil convention. From the stage we noticed a large crowd of Fianna Fáil delegates wearing colourful rosettes gathering at the bar. It took half an hour of loud rock and roll before they twigged that the De Valera whose gig they were attending was a rock singer and not a member of Ireland's illustrious political family.

We played the Arcadia in Cork. Some girls sang along to our

songs, a sure sign that we were doing it right. Once girls started going to a band's gigs, it was only a matter of time before that band made it. It was the first law of rock. A few more gigs like tonight's and we would be up there with The Boomtown Rats.

Backstage I tried to impress a local girl by telling her that I had a degree in English. She laughed so hard that I thought she was going to strangle herself. 'Rocky De Valera has a degree in English,' she choked. 'Now I've heard everything.'

On the way home from Cork, the van spluttered to a halt on a dark stretch of road. We piled out, tired and sore but still high on the adrenalin of playing a live gig to a large audience. 'I'm not sure what's wrong, but I definitely think I can fix it,' the driver said.

While the driver got to work on the van, someone produced a football and we played a soccer match in the middle of the road by moonlight. Luckily there was no traffic. Playing football on the road in the dark was daft as well as dangerous, but it was a lot better than sitting in a freezing van.

When the van started chugging again, we grabbed the ball and climbed back inside. We made slow but steady progress for a few miles before the engine cut out again.

'It's all right,' the driver said. 'We're only two hundred miles from Dublin.'

★

I decided that we needed to get ourselves on a professional footing. We found a roadie – Woodstock – who had long hair and a great laugh. He looked after our stage gear and handled the sound desk.

We played several gigs in McGonagles. We did interviews on pirate stations and were interviewed by several underground magazines.

We played the Project Arts Centre at midnight. During the

first number I twirled the microphone over my head like a lasso. The microphone flew off the lead and into the audience, braining some hippy. We had to stop so that I could ask for the microphone back.

On the way home, the police stopped our van. A hefty cop approached the driver's window. He wanted to know who was inside. We told him we were Rocky De Valera and the Gravediggers coming back from a gig. He cracked up and called his colleague over and asked us to repeat the name of the band. The other cop cracked up too. We gave them a poster and they told us we were free to go.

We played a lunchtime charity gig in the Bridgefoot Street Adventure Playground. The makeshift stage wobbled so badly that the drums kept falling over. Afterwards Dave and I argued about the gig. He said that the Bridgefoot Street gig should never have been agreed to. There was no proper stage, someone could have been hurt and we were playing to tiny kids.

I knew that he was right, but I refused to admit it. I accused him of being unprofessional. A week later we made up, but relations between us remained strained.

A bunch of us went to see U2 play a new venue, the Celebrity Club in Abbey Street. They played a loud, fast set and there was a small but enthusiastic audience. I noticed that Bono and The Edge were wearing strange, colourful jumpers that almost matched, as though someone had knitted them specially.

At one point, The Edge leapt off the stage to play guitar from the audience. A big space cleared around him. After a few moments, The Edge glanced back at Bono. 'Get back up here now,' Bono scowled. The Edge climbed back on stage without dropping a note.

We played a gig in the Howth Community Centre, with support from The Modulators and Ireland's first all-girl punk group, The Boy Scoutz. I fancied Catwoman, the guitarist from The Boy Scoutz, but my old shyness kicked in. For some reason, I couldn't get it together to do more than exchange a few words with her. Her beauty intimidated me. When I tried to ask her out, my mouth felt like it was filled with crab apples and I gave up.

It turned out to be a great gig. U2 came to watch us from the side of the stage. Catwoman played great guitar and looked better than Gaye Advert, the much-lusted-after bassist from The Adverts.

That weekend Larry, U2's drummer, phoned me at home. He congratulated me again on a great night and asked me for the name of the promoter. U2 wanted to play the community centre but Larry didn't want to gatecrash. He hoped that I didn't have a problem with that because he knew that we were the first ones to play the venue. Not at all, I said and gave him the phone number of the promoter. He thanked me again and wished me luck for the future. I put the phone down thinking that Larry was the best-mannered person I had ever met, in rock and roll or anywhere.

We were booked to play the Celebrity Club. We turned up and did a really good sound check. We forgot to put up posters, but we assured the owner that word of mouth would guarantee us a good crowd, bigger than the audience who came to see U2.

Nobody showed up for the gig so the club owner cancelled it. That put everyone in bad form. I left the Celebrity Club feeling embarrassed and lost. I couldn't manage the band alone, I didn't know what I was doing. We needed a professional manager to sort out bookings and money and posters and all the rest of the crap.

Pat met me for a drink in Slattery's and offered his services as manager. I turned him down. I wanted him as my friend, not my manager. I could see that I'd hurt him and had to backtrack quickly. 'Wait a little while,' I told him. 'If we can't get a professional, experienced rock manager within the next month, then you can have the gig.'

That only made things worse. We drank our pints in silence. 'I'd make a great manager,' Pat said. 'You don't know what you're missing.'

★

We recorded a demo in small studio in Balinteer, but it sounded terrible. The results were not worth the few hundred quid we'd managed to cobble together to pay for it. Our version of Buddy Holly's 'Midnight Shift' sounded particularly wretched. The sound engineer told me that the song was about a prostitute. That surprised me – I had presumed it was about a girl who worked late. 'Same difference,' the sound engineer replied.

We met Bart, a friend of a friend. He had never managed a band before, but he knew about business and was willing to invest money. A lot of money. He was willing to buy us our own van and amplifiers and everything we needed. He was willing to look into getting us a permanent rehearsal space. Maybe he would rent a big house. He told us we were a great band. He said I was a superb motivator. There was talk of setting up a tour of England and more talk of going to meet with Stiff Records.

I grew excited, convinced that Bart was the right man to manage us. I offered him the job and he accepted.

However, he did have some thoughts.

Bart told me that it would be a good idea to drop the 'De Valera' from the band's name. The band had already made an impact and no longer needed to employ 'shock tactics'. Besides, Rocky and the Gravediggers was a much neater, cleaner name for a band. Bart had discovered from asking around that promoters were reluctant to book us because of the De Valera tag. The punk thing was dead so it made sense to lose the famous surname altogether. It also meant that the Irish press would have no excuse to deliberately keep misspelling the name of the band – in the gig guides, the press usually referred to us as, among other things, 'Rocky Malaria' and 'Rocky Valerie' or even 'Rocky Marciano and the Ravedraggers'. Bart also asked me to think about dropping some of the louder, faster numbers. People wanted melodic songs, he said. All we had to do was to agree to change the name of the band and alter the style of music we played and he would manage us.

Reluctantly, I agreed to lose the De Valera tag. It felt like lopping off a limb.

Within a week, new posters arrived for Rocky and the Gravediggers. The band decided that they didn't want to play twelve-bar songs anymore. They wanted to do more musical songs, songs that had more than three chords. They felt we should do more harmonies.

Something wasn't quite right. We had changed line-ups several times and now we were losing part of our identity and were thinking of changing musical direction. I tried to get everyone motivated again, but things became strained. I began to drive people mad. I began to drive myself mad.

At a sound check in McGonagles, I went upstairs to talk to someone. As I made my way back to the stage, I noticed the drummer and Dave Hero in a huddle. When they saw me coming they broke apart and looked guilty – I didn't think anything of it. The gig was OK. Someone said that CBS were in the audience but nothing came of it. I couldn't understand why record companies weren't interested in signing us. We were approaching our peak. Bart wasn't doing his job.

Before taking the stage in McGonagles, we went across the street for drinks in Larry Tobin's. Outside the pub I ran into Kim, a beautiful girl with big brown eyes I'd known for years, and asked her if she was going to the gig. She sighed. 'I really like you, Ferdia,' she said. 'But I just can't stand your band's music. I've tried to like it, but I don't and I'm really sorry.'

We played a terrible gig. Strings broke. Feedback and whistles haunted the PA system. We drew a small, drunken crowd who constantly heckled us.

A few days after the McGonagles gig, Bart called a band meeting downstairs in the Bruxelles. I travelled in by bus from Howth with Big Jack. We arrived at Bruxelles ten minutes early to find the others already there. The others had sombre faces, like they were about to go to a funeral. For some reason they wouldn't let Jack or me sit on the empty chairs alongside them. They said there was no room, so we sat opposite.

Bart told me that he was pulling out. He didn't think there was anything further he could do for the band. I was shocked, but also relieved. This meant we could get a proper manager and restore 'De Valera' to the band's name.

Then Dave said that he was quitting too. Then the drummer said that he was out as well. The rhythm guitarist also quit. They had had enough. They thought the band had gone as far as it was likely to go.

I sat there beside Big Jack and pretended that the news had not affected me too much. I put on a front. I told them that they would be sorry. I would just get new guys in. I tried to block out the thought that the band was finished. I tried to block out the notion that this coup had been brewing for some time. I tried not to break into tears.

Dave had quit. I felt that the guy I started the band with had betrayed me. I couldn't understand it. I hated Dave. I wished I'd thrown him out instead. I didn't care about the others. I wished I'd never hired Bart. I wished I'd taken it a bit easier on everyone.

Now there was just myself and Big Jack.

Jack and I left and walked around for a while. We might have gone for a drink in The Bailey. The afternoon was a scorcher and the sunlight made Grafton Street seem like a street in sunny California. It didn't seem like Dublin. People shimmered in a heat haze in the distance. How could my band break up on a beautiful day like that?

That night Jack and I met in The Cock Tavern in Howth for a drink with friends. I felt very alone and lost but tried not to show it. Jack remained upbeat. 'We'll hold auditions,' he said. 'We'll get new players. We'll make it big this time.'

At midnight we drove around Howth Strand in someone's car, listening to Zappa and Dr Feelgood tapes. The driver did mad twists and turns at speed, spewing up sand storms behind us. I think he was trying to cheer me up.

I felt heartbroken. No amount of optimistic talk or high japes could change my mood. I saw the break-up, and particularly Dave quitting, as the end of a dream. I felt like a total failure. I didn't seem to have any strength in my arms or hands and my stomach churned like it was feeding on itself. Booze had no effect on me. I had never felt more disillusioned or more sober. It was the worst feeling I had ever had.

I was out of college and was about to leave the flat in Rathmines because I couldn't afford the rent. I had let go of my job on the badges stall in the Dandelion. After the band fell apart I blamed myself, but I hated Dave as well. Why hadn't he discussed it with me first? Maybe I had driven the others mad.

But the band had something. The band had magic.

The next day I met Pat in Rathmines and we went for breakfast in a small diner on the main street. He had heard about the band and was really sorry. We had been really good. What was I going to do now?

I told him that I was going to get a new band together. 'Maybe I'll call this one Rocky De Valera and the Gangsters.'

Pat stopped and gave me a big smile. 'I'm glad,' he said.

We finished breakfast and Pat led me into the supermarket where he had 'borrowed' the rashers and eggs a few months earlier. He went to the girl at the cash register and counted out some money that he then handed to her. He told her that he had 'accidentally' forgotten to pay for some items a little while back and wanted to pay for them now. Surprised the girl accepted the money. Pat gave her a big smile and we walked out. 'I said I'd go back, didn't I?' he said.

That night I got a phone call from Fiona, my ex. She said that she was sorry to hear about my band. I told her that I was putting another group together. This one would be better than the last. 'You know, you don't have to do this,' she said. 'There are a lot of other things you could do.'

Later, after I put the phone down, I thought about my life and the way things had worked out. I was about to turn twenty-three. I had no job, no flat and was back living at home with my parents. Perhaps putting a new band together would be tilting against the natural order of things. Maybe I should just forget rock and roll. Fiona was right. There were other things I could do.

Like get a job.

Like rejoin Planet Normal.

Like punch Dave Hero in the nose.

★

We held auditions in our garage in Howth. Mother brought us plates of sausages and toast and didn't ask me about college. My mother was very supportive. Dad wanted to know when I was going to look for a job.

Gradually, I came back to life. We went through a number of guitarists before finding Martin, a quiet guy from Finglas who could play rockabilly and blues and rock and roll. We called him The Lizard because of the lizard-skin guitar strap he wore.

We found a drummer and rehearsed new songs. We kept

some of the old numbers like 'Brand New Cadillac', 'Red Hot' and 'Little Piece of Leather' and I dug up new songs by obscure rockabilly acts such as Sid King and the Five Strings, Jimmy Heap and Charlie Feathers, as well as contemporary Welsh Rockabillies, Crazy Cavan and The Rhythm Rockers.

The new band rehearsed in our garage, driving the neighbours insane. Hordes of small kids from the area sat on the banks of our driveway or hung around the back fields to listen to our rehearsals.

As a four-piece, we started playing gigs. Our first was a comeback gig in Howth Community Centre. We were so naïve we forgot to put someone on the door to count the takings. We filled the place, but only ended up with enough money to pay for the posters and hired amps and we only took home two pounds fifty each. The money didn't matter – the money never mattered to me – we had made a comeback and that was the important thing. It was always crucial to keep things in perspective. That was what I told the others in the band when they gave out shite about only getting two pounds fifty. They didn't like it, but they accepted it. They suggested that we should get ourselves a manager. Reluctantly, I agreed. 'We'll hold auditions,' I said.

Afterwards the band and friends brought some beers back to my house in Howth. Mother was very understanding. Some French people arrived at the door, but nobody knew them so we didn't let them inside. They got very upset and vowed to get revenge. People slept on the floor in the living room or conked out in the study. Nobody was allowed to sleep on Dad's black leather chair.

The next morning, Dad took a look around at all the sleeping bodies. 'I have learned one thing in life,' he said. 'If your son decides to call himself Rocky De Valera and start a rock band, then let him.'

Later I travelled into town to get more badges and posters. Painted in large letters on the wall at Sutton Strand was the sentence, '*Rocky De Valera est un wimp absolutement.*'

A week later Rocker called out to Howth to say goodbye. Hero had joined The Vipers and they were touring England with The Boomtown Rats. Rocker had been invited along as the roadie. I wished him good luck, but inside I felt betrayed again. I felt as though I had a walk-on part in a movie where I should have been the star.

★

We were booked to play Trinity Junior Common Room as support to Joe Jackson, a rising new-wave singer and songwriter, who complimented our attitude when he came on stage. After the gig, he invited us to his dressing room for a drink, so we went. We got on well and Joe and I had a good chat and promised to keep in touch.

Pat bought me a farewell pint – he was off to London to manage a pool hall. I told him I'd see him in London when we played the Hammersmith Odeon or The Marquee.

Somehow we ended up with a new manager, Doggie, though none of us could remember hiring him. Doggie was a genial guy who ran gigs in Finglas. He didn't seem like a jet setter, but we trusted him. Plus he was a fan of the band, and at that stage being a big fan made him ideally qualified for the job.

Along with The Virgin Prunes, Nigel Rolfe and many others, we played the Dark Space gig at The Project, twenty-four hours of continuous music, performance art and other events. John Peel gave the band a good review in *Sounds.* We were up there with Revolver. My confidence returned and I began to become deluded again about our chances of making it big.

Doggie got us a residency in Toner's of Baggot Street and persuaded Terri Hooley of Good Vibrations Records in Belfast to front the money for us to record a four-track single for the label. We recorded four original songs in Lombard Studios and gave one song to a new Irish sampler album, *Just for Kicks*.

Doggie showed me his manager's accounts book. He had written 'The Bread Story' on the cover. Inside, every page was blank. 'Give it time,' Doggie said.

Doggie and I travelled to Belfast on the Express to hand over the master tapes, but we left them on the train and had to stop it to reclaim them. People thought it was a bomb scare and the police told us not to be so careless in future.

Later Terri Hooley bought us pints in the Harp Bar. The Outcasts were playing and I was asked up to sing with them. Following hurried discussions on stage, we eventually staggered through a twisted, gnarly version of 'Good Golly Miss Molly'.

Afterwards Terri Hooley was ecstatic. 'Getting up on stage here tonight means that you have sold at least a hundred copies of your single. These people will remember you.'

We watched The Outcasts play. Aggressive, sharp and exciting – they were a great band.

Just before the encore something plopped into my beer. I looked down to see a glass eye swirling around. 'Didn't expect that, did you?' Terri Hooley said and retrieved his glass eye. He wiped it and then popped it back into his socket.

★

A couple of mornings later I woke with a chronic toothache. Mother made an appointment with a really good dentist in Clontarf, Mr Ryan, father of my sister's friend, Gerry Ryan the radio DJ.

I took a taxi to Clontarf and sat in the dentist's chair in my jeans and leather jacket as Mr Ryan went to work on my tooth. He kept calling me Ferdia, which upset me.

When he finished giving my tooth a filling, I stood up, washed my mouth out and shook his hand. Then he called me Ferdia again.

I decided I couldn't let this continue. 'The name is Rocky,' I told him. 'Rocky De Valera.'

13

I Was Gay Byrne's Banana

Gay Byrne was small, trim and confident. The most famous television star in Ireland strode into the canteen briskly. Arriving at the booth where I was seated, he gave me a smart handshake and then sat opposite. He wore a strange yellow tie that seemed to have been made out of a banana.

It was summer 1978 and I had applied for two jobs in RTÉ – the first as a radio producer and the second as a researcher in television programmes. I had been through several stages of formal interviews and sat for various IQ tests and all the rest, but I had heard nothing.

I presumed that I had failed to impress.

That morning I had received a phone call from someone in personnel. Could I be at the canteen in RTÉ at three that afternoon? Gay Byrne wanted to talk to me about a confidential matter. 'Fine,' I said.

I had arrived in the main canteen in RTÉ shortly before

three to find the place deserted except for staff. I was anxious about meeting Gay. I had seen the *Late Late* over the years but I had never been a fan. Dad had appeared on the show several times, usually in connection with the latest Abbey drama. I regarded it as a two-hours-plus mix of chat and controversy interspersed with dreary light entertainment that older people watched.

I didn't care for light entertainment and had made no secret of that in my interviews. I didn't want to be shanghaied into doing something that was against my principles – whatever they were. I saw the *Late Late* as a slow death after the anarchy of college and the buzz of rock and roll.

Yet here I was sitting opposite Gay Byrne, Ireland's most influential and famous TV personality, presumably about to be interviewed for a job. I had to fight hard to keep my gaze off his weird yellow tie.

Gay asked me if I would like to work on *The Late Late Show*. I decided to be honest. I told him that I wasn't really interested. The *Late Late* was not my kind of thing. But he didn't seem worried by my answer.

He asked if I would have any objection to giving up Saturday nights to work on one of the world's last remaining live prime-time talk shows. I said that I would rather be out with my friends on a Saturday night.

He wondered if I would be excited by working in a live television environment. I told him that I had no interest in live TV.

'Great,' Gay said. 'You've got the job. You start on Tuesday.'

He gave me a big smile, shook my hand and then he strode decisively out of the canteen, leaving me confused as well as intrigued.

I wondered if he had heard anything I had said. He had scarcely looked me in the eye once, a significant feat considering that he had been seated directly opposite me. The Great Interviewer had asked me three questions and received what should have been disappointing answers. I had informed the host of the country's top TV show that I had no interest in working with him – yet he gave me the job anyway.

Television was a peculiar business.

★

My girlfriend Jenny was puzzled. She asked me to explain again about the *Late Late* job offer. We sat in the kitchen of our small flat in Clontarf while I went over the story once more. 'So you turned down the job and then he hired you?' she asked.

All I could do was nod. She told me that I might as well take it. 'You've got nothing to lose,' she said.

I was still singing with the band. Rocky De Valera and the Gravediggers played gigs around Dublin. We had built up a sizeable cult following, still playing the Sunday night residency in the basement of Toner's of Baggot Street. Sundays could be wild. We attracted all sorts, from bikers to teenyboppers as well as gangsters.

We also attracted people who fell into no known category. 'My brother loves you guys,' a tall, wild-eyed biker told us one Sunday night. 'He gets out next week so he's coming to see yis.' The biker's eyes grew even wider. 'And he's bringing his mates.'

The Gravediggers were impressed by my job offer, but they were concerned that my 'going legit' might spell the end of the band. I told them I could still work and rock.

They didn't believe me. I was determined not to give up the band. Working in RTÉ would compliment my career as a rocker. I was convinced that I could do both. Deep down, I was relieved that I would finally be getting a regular wage. I wondered what it would be like to live a normal, settled-down life. I figured that I would do the *Late Late* gig until the radio producer job came up. In my heart, I knew that the band would end soon.

I showed up in RTÉ on the following Tuesday. Someone gave me directions to the *Late Late* offices, which were inside a large rectangular annex that looked like an oversized porta-kabin. An attractive young blonde woman called Ces answered the door. She welcomed me to the team.

Inside, the office was cramped and stale smelling. I was surprised that a successful prime-time live talk show and RTÉ's flagship for over twenty years was housed inside a dingy caravan.

I was the replacement for a researcher who was moving to a new career in radio as a producer. The previous guy had an excellent reputation. It was made clear to me that I would be stepping into a big pair of boots.

Gay sat at a table at the top of the long room. I was surprised to find that he was so accessible. I had presumed that he would have his own suite of offices somewhere.

He didn't seem to need to have his ego constantly massaged, though he did seem somewhat removed from ordinary office banter. Nor did he seem like the kind of guy who would be inclined to go for a pint with the team after a show – or any time, for that matter.

In the first couple of weeks I noticed that Gay was patient as long as a person was trying, but he could be abrupt and even rude if he suspected slacking off or lazy research. 'I don't think much of your item for *The Late Late Show*, Mr Mac Anna,' he said in front of everyone after I pitched my first idea.

I had suggested that we showcase a bunch of Irish Hell's Angels on the show. 'We can have them drive on from the scene dock in single file and then line up their Harley Davidsons in the performance area,' I had enthused, eliciting complete silence from the team.

Nobody had interviewed Irish Hell's Angels on TV before. Perhaps the idea was just ahead of its time – or maybe it was just a crap idea. It was decided that the idea needed more work.

The Tuesday postmortem meetings were often cut-throat. Items that hadn't worked on the previous Saturday night were ruthlessly dissected and the researcher responsible was held to account without feelings being spared. Once the previous week's show had been settled, the agenda switched to the coming Saturday night's show. That was where the real jousting began.

During my first season, the *Late Late* team comprised Gay (who was his own producer), Adrian (the show's long-time director), Collette (the programme PA), Maura (the programme secretary), senior researcher Pan Collins (who had actually been with the show longer than Gay, who had left and been replaced by Frank Hall for several months in the early sixties) and up to six researchers, including Howard, who befriended me and helped me settle in.

At the meetings – in fact, throughout the week leading up to the show – researchers competed to get Gay's approval for their ideas. Gay always listened to what people had to say. He would entertain any idea, no matter how daft it seemed initially, if he thought that it might make a good item on the show. He was always ready for a good debate or argument.

Most of the ideas for items and guests came from the researchers, but everyone was expected to chip in and give their opinions and ideas. The meetings could be fraught, yet there was rarely any bad blood afterwards. The programme had a simple premise: whatever was deemed to be good for the show got on air. Not whatever was good for RTÉ or the country or even Gay Byrne. Flattery and bullshit got you nowhere.

Gay himself was often severely criticised by the team if they felt that he had failed to do justice to an item or an interview with a guest. If he thought that the criticism was justified, he took it on the chin.

Gay took a lot of flak over his dress sense. He showed up at one Tuesday meeting wearing a loud purple and orange jumper that looked like a nuclear incident. He had intended to wear it for the following week's Toy Show. He asked the team what they thought of his choice and we told him. 'There's nothing wrong with this jumper,' he protested. 'It's brand new.'

Another Saturday night, he proudly sported a mauve tie that had tiny coloured dots all over it, as though thousands of insects had chosen its surface upon which to commit hara-kiri. He always seemed amazed at any critique of his clothing. He never thought that there was a problem.

Eventually the criticism wore him down, and on air he would wear clothing that, if not stylish, was at least suited to his shape and colouring – though a good percentage of the time he stuck to his usual fashion atrocities.

★

Shortly after I joined the show, I noticed that some people seemed to have trouble getting their heads around my name. I received mail addressed to 'Fernando Bandana' and 'Feruka Manana'. Once I received a letter for 'Mac Bono'.

My colleagues enjoyed handing me letters where my name was mangled and misspelled, but they also enjoyed holding up the telephone receiver to say, 'Call for Mr Banana.'

My first assignment was to set up an interview with a group of Jesuit priests, who were committed to helping the poor and who were about to head for the Philippines to do missionary work. They weren't just interested in saving souls, they wanted to help the living as well, especially the disenfranchised and the impoverished who had been marginalised by the military regime of Marcos. That brought them into conflict with the authorities and gave their work a political hue.

On the night, the priest that I had selected for interview spoke passionately – it also helped that he looked like Robert Redford. The item went down well, but the audience had responded to the appealing persona of the handsome priest rather than the radical message he was preaching that effective missionary work had by necessity to be political.

Afterwards a quiet, bespectacled priest who had taken part in the audience discussion took me aside to tell me that he had been to the Philippines several times and had slept with women. He believed that it was unnatural that Catholic priests should be celibate. He said that priests should be allowed to marry, a belief shared by many of his fellow priests. He wanted to know if that shocked me. I told him that it didn't. I wondered if he would be willing to go on the *Late Late* and be interviewed about it. 'You must be fucking joking,' he laughed. 'I still have to come back to this country to visit my mother.'

That night my name was included on the *Late Late* list of researchers on the roller at the top of the show. My name would remain featured until I left the programme. I felt good about seeing my name go out into the world. It made me feel that I was normal – for the time being, at any rate.

My role in the team was to come up with items or guests that would appeal to young people, that is, anyone between the ages of fifteen and thirty-five. The *Late Late* was the number one show in television and had been for many years, but it was considered important to build viewer loyalty with younger viewers, especially those who were disdainful of the stuffy old *Late Late* and of its conservative presenter.

One night I asked Gay why he had hired me. He told me that he been impressed by my honesty as well as by my apparent lack of enthusiasm for the live talk-show format and for the *Late Late*. He had reasoned that if I didn't like the show, I would try to change it and if I tried to change it, a dynamic would be created that would be good for the show. He liked to have diversity on the team. A bunch of yes men would be unlikely to contribute engaging or radical ideas. He had given me the opportunity to show what I could do. Now it was up to me.

I was flattered that he didn't consider me a yes man, but I wasn't sure if I could fulfil the role he had earmarked for me. I didn't share the passion for the programme that some of my fellow researchers had. I felt like an outsider. The other researchers were devoted to the show, forever coming up with ideas of items and guests that would appeal to the public. I came up with youth items or the occasional cult novelist or off-the-wall guests.

Ubi Dwyer, for example, was a hospital worker who had gotten into trouble with the authorities because he liked to dress up and carry on like a priest. He had built up a sizeable following and gained some notoriety. I had to fight hard to get him on the show. Perhaps because he was so eccentric and harmless seeming, Ubi went down well.

I identified more with some of the crank characters than with the stream of successful entrepreneurs and showbiz types that were featured on the show. I didn't think successful people were terribly interesting and most success stories sounded the same. I preferred the oddballs or the nonconformists or those who had a human-interest story to tell.

Nevertheless, it was a thrill to be a member of an exclusive crew. *The Late Late Show* basically operated as an independent unit within RTÉ. The team didn't mix with other programmes. In the late seventies, Ireland was still basically in two-channel land – RTÉ 1 and RTÉ 2. The *Late Late* was a huge attraction and it was uncategorisable, neither pure entertainment nor current affairs nor traditional talk show. On the *Late Late* anything could happen. That unpredictability, whereby guests or items were never advertised ahead of transmission, gave the show a unique appeal and kept it at the top.

I was sent to interview Cyril Cusack for a possible special on his life in the theatre. We met in his dressing room in the Abbey shortly before a performance of *The Vicar of Wakefield*. He was dressed as a bishop. Instead of shaking hands he held out his hand for me to kiss his ring. I shook his ring hand and sat down, pretending not to notice that he was 'in character'. He asked me what they wanted with him out in RTÉ and I told him that the *Late Late* wanted to do a special interview with him. 'Oh, I couldn't do that now, dear boy. Come back and see me next year.' He waved his ring, turned to his dressing-room mirror and the interview was over.

After a show one night, Maura told me that Gay was an artist. Inwardly I sneered at her assessment of Gay's talents. How could a TV presenter be an artist? He was an excellent professional and that was all. Maura could tell that I was sceptical. 'There are lots of TV presenters who can interview people,' she continued in her quiet voice. 'But very few of them ever listen to what the guests are saying. The thing about Gay is that he listens.'

I pretended to see her point, but I wasn't convinced. Gay was the best talk-show host we had, but that didn't put him up there with Van Gogh or De Niro or Phil Lynott. (Looking back at it all now, I feel that Maura had a point. Gay took his work as seriously as any artist. He set himself high standards and he lived up to them.)

*

In 1978 I was sent to London by RTÉ for three weeks to research a *Late Late Show* special that would be broadcast live – it was the first time I'd been in London since my college days. My specific role was to assist the senior researcher, Garvan, who had just joined the team. Garvan was a hands-on guy. He liked to be totally on top of what he was doing. He didn't need some young fella getting in his face.

I ended up with a lot of free time so I decided to look up some old friends. I called Joey, but he couldn't come to the phone. Later I called to his house in Wood Green, but the relative who answered the door said he was sick and couldn't leave his bedroom. Nobody except family was allowed to visit him in his room.

I called Marvo, but he was busy. He told me that Joey had quit working to 'retire indoors'. He said Joey was in good form. I got the impression that something bad had happened to Joey in the bakery, but I couldn't find out anything specific.

Fiona and I had split up years earlier. Our last date had been at a first night at the Abbey Theatre to see some crap play. We had broken up during the intermission. She had been the love of my young life, but I was too restless and troubled and all over the place to settle down with her. I hurt her when I broke it off, but I had been unhappy and I had given her a rough time. I still missed her from time to time, but I never did anything about it. At the time I was living in a small apartment on the northside of Dublin with Jenny, a woman that I didn't love anymore. We were good friends and had an open relationship – which basically boiled down to each of us going off with or having flings with whoever we chose. What we were doing together was a mystery, but it seemed to suit us at the time.

On my day off, I travelled to Rock On Records of Camden Town. I wanted to find a record I liked, *Sweet Dreams* by Tommy McLain. I couldn't find the album in the racks when, at that moment, the song began to play on the store's sound system. I went to the counter to investigate. A tall, skinny woman in a short skirt and leather top was standing at the counter listening to the music while she examined the record sleeve. In her hands she held the cover for *Sweet Dreams*.

I got talking to her. My shyness usually disappeared around music. Her name was Stella and she loved Cajun music. I told her that it was rare to find anyone who liked Cajun stuff – or 'swamp pop' as Tommy McLain's brand of balladry was sometimes known. She bought the Tommy McLain, which was the last copy in the shop. I told her that I didn't mind, she had got there first. Before she left I asked for her phone number. She wrote it on the front of her *New Musical Express* and handed the paper to me.

The next morning I called her. Would she like to come to see Nine Below Zero at the Marquee? 'That's very sweet of you,' she said. 'I would be delighted.'

She asked me where I was staying. She said she hated public transport and taxis. She had a car, so if I had no objections she'd pick me up outside my hotel at seven. I had no objections.

At seven, I was standing outside the hotel when a sleek E-Type Jaguar pulled in to the kerb. Stella gave me a big smile. Sweet Dreams was playing in the cassette player. She had taped it especially so that we could listen to it while we were driving around. I climbed in and she sped off into the London traffic. Sitting in the passenger seat of an E-Type jag with music blaring and a beautiful woman driving, I felt a bit like a kept man. I was surprised to find that it was not an unpleasant sensation.

Nine Below Zero were loud and fast and exhilarating, but they were just a better than average R&B band, nothing special. Afterwards we drove around London for a while. We took slugs of gin from her silver hip flask.

She took me back to her apartment on Tottenham Court Road. We chose albums from her record collection and played them on an elaborate, pearl-panelled record player. She told me she'd had the record player specially made.

Stella had worked in television and movies. She was a lot older than me. She showed me pictures of her younger self. She had always been a beauty, but she was much skinnier and prettier now. She told me that she had left that world behind her because of too many 'false people'. 'I used to be really somebody,' she said without a trace of wistfulness. 'But I'm much more content now, or at least I soon will be.'

She said that she didn't know what she wanted to do with her life, but that she could afford not to worry about it for a while. She was the Queen of Tottenham Court Road, hadn't I realised? I said that I definitely had.

There was something odd about Stella, but I liked that. I liked the fact that she was different. She didn't seem to be worried about what anyone thought of her, yet at the same time there was a definite vulnerability to her. I got the impression that she was only now emerging from some trauma. I wasn't surprised when she leaned over and kissed me. We stayed on the sofa for a while, kissing and messing around.

Then she broke away. 'You'll probably want to have sex with me now, won't you?' she said matter-of-factly. Before I could answer she took my hand and led me to the bedroom, which was covered in red and blue velvet. There were no windows. Instead a huge painted drape hung opposite the bed showing a scene from the court of Queen Cleopatra. She told me to get into bed. She said that she hated light and switched off the lamps. Then she left the bedroom. I stripped except for my underpants and climbed into bed. The sheets felt like silk. Stella was gone for ages. After a long time, the bedroom door opened and she slipped in beside me. We made love. The sex was enjoyable but detached, as though Stella was going through the motions. Maybe she was scared of becoming too intimate.

In the morning, she was gone. I got up quickly and dressed. I felt uncomfortable and exposed. I wanted to get out of Stella's velvet palace.

I found Stella by the front door in a dressing gown. She was wrapping a red ribbon around the Tommy McLain album. She had attached a note saying, 'With love, The Queen of Tottenham Court Road'. I thanked her and we kissed. I left with the album under my arm, feeling like a young God.

I met Marvo that night in a pub in Soho. He turned up with a strange expression on his face. He seemed so odd and out of it that it was difficult to make conversation. I was drinking Coke, but for some reason he kept buying me gin and tonics. When I asked him to quit buying me gins, he looked at me slyly as though I were letting him in on a private joke. 'Nice one,' he said, and immediately went to the bar to buy me a gin and tonic.

Later we got talking to two girls at the next table. Marvo seemed keen to chat them up, even though their boyfriends were standing close by. Marvo appeared perfectly normal, until he suddenly leaned forward to leer at one of the women.

'I'd love to eat your pussy,' he said loudly enough for everyone in the pub to hear.

There was a stunned silence. The boyfriends moved towards us. Then the girl laughed. 'Oh shut up, you idiot,' she said, momentarily diffusing the tension.

However, the boyfriends glared at us with a mean look on their faces. Marvo didn't behave as though he sensed anything amiss. The boyfriends were big guys – very big guys.

I grabbed Marvo and steered him towards the door. I apologised for my friend. I told them he was a bit out of it. Once I got Marvo outside I ran, pulling him with me. Behind me I heard the door of the pub opening, but I didn't dare to look around.

Once we were clear of the pub, I hailed a taxi and we went back to my hotel. At the hotel Marvo ordered more drinks. A colleague from the *Late Late* team joined us, but Marvo took offence to the way he was dressed.

'Look at his poncey clobber,' he shouted.

Suddenly, Marvo turned on my colleague and grabbed him by the throat. I pulled Marvo off and told him to take it easy. 'Get away from these civil service pricks,' Marvo said. 'They will destroy your mind.'

After Marvo was rude to the porter and several other guests, I led him out of the hotel and onto the street. We walked towards the lights of the West End. Marvo grabbed a lantern from a road works and walked with it on his head. He kept the lantern on his head even after a police car pulled in alongside us. 'You guys are always spoiling my fun,' Marvo told the policemen.

I did a lot of talking. I explained that my friend was the worse for wear and I was seeing him home. The police left after we promised to put the lantern back where Marvo had found it.

We walked to the West End. I was confused and hurt by Marvo's behaviour. I hadn't seen him for years and now he had turned up to our first meeting out of his skull on something. I couldn't understand why anyone would behave like that. I took it personally, as though the thought of a few hours in my company was enough to cause even an old friend to reach for a mind-altering substance.

Marvo refused a taxi and insisted that he could make his own way home. He had lost his keys but they would show up. He said that he would go and stay with Janet, even though he hadn't seen her in years. He waved and wandered off, leaving me standing shocked and bewildered in the middle of Piccadilly Circus. That was the last time I saw Marvo.

My special role as researcher on the London show was to ensure that the Irish soccer star Liam Brady, who had just published his autobiography, made it to the TV studio on time.

The show was being broadcast live. Arsenal was playing a European Cup second-leg tie, but as they had won the away leg already they were expected to trash their opponents easily. That would mean that Brady would be substituted early and be free to leave the grounds before the match was over, thus avoiding the crowds. I had approximately forty minutes to get Brady from Arsenal's ground at Highbury to the TV studios on the other side of the Thames. Brady refused the offer of a driver, saying that he would drive himself. I was welcome to come with him.

I arrived just after kickoff. An elderly porter showed me to a seat in the stands. Arsenal led 3–1 within half an hour. Brady scored a fourth just after half-time and was immediately substituted. The porter tapped me on the shoulder and led me through a long, impressively marbled passageway and through a side door to an outside car park, where Brady had already changed and was waiting in his car. I climbed in and we drove to the TV studios. I had been expecting to meet an arrogant superstar, but Brady was a straightforward and down-to-earth Dublin guy. He didn't have much to say, but he was polite and easy-going. I wondered what kind of impression he would make on the *Late Late*. I figured that the audience would respond well to his lack of pretension and guile. I reckoned that they would accept him as one of their own made good and not some talented chancer who had made a name for himself across the water.

Crossing London Bridge a car in front of us hit another car. 'Will you look at this,' Brady said. For a moment it looked as though there was going to be a massive pile-up at speed. However, the drivers in front of us retained control of their cars and Brady swerved at the right moment. 'That was too close,' he said.

We made it to the TV studios where the *Late Late* was going out live. Brady parked and was immediately whisked off to make-up. Ten minutes after arriving at the studio, he was being interviewed by Gay Byrne – and he went down well with the audience.

The London *Late Late* was interesting, but it wasn't one of the most riveting shows. The big discussion on Northern Ireland failed to catch fire, despite the contribution of RTÉ's London correspondent John O'Callaghan, who had made the point that if the IRA wanted to get people talking about Northern Ireland all they had to do was put a bomb in a Tube train. Nobody seemed to want to talk about terrorist tactics or aims.

Afterwards Gay said he was happy with the show. He said that the discussion about Northern Ireland should have had a bit more flavour. Maybe people were sick of discussing the North. 'Well done, son,' he said to Garvan. Garvan grimaced. He hated when Gay called him 'son'. He had just been offered a new job in news. He told me that he was delighted to be leaving the *Late Late*.

The day after the London *Late Late* was my last in the city. I went to see Stella in her apartment. I brought her a Nine Below Zero album as a present.

We listened to music for a while. Then we kissed for a short time. I made a move to unbutton her top. She gently stayed my hand. 'Must we?' she said softly. 'Can't we just cuddle and listen to great music?'

So we cuddled and listened to great music instead. I felt my interest in Stella slipping away.

Later that night we exchanged addresses and contact numbers and made plans to meet and ticked off all of the motions that people go through when they have no intention of ever meeting each other again.

The next morning before leaving for the airport, I phoned Joey. A woman's voice told me that he couldn't come to the phone.

★

Before I joined, I had presumed that Gay was a conservative fuddy-duddy. I was surprised that he liked to get his hands dirty. As his own producer, Gay fought the management of the station for the right to be allowed to tackle the controversial issues of the day or take on subjects that might get RTÉ into difficulty with the politicians or the far right or the Church. He usually won the battles with the bureaucrats and managers who ran RTÉ, though he once famously lost his bid to interview a pair of lesbian nuns. As far as I'm aware, that was the only setback he suffered during my two seasons on the show.

Section 31 was an Irish government directive that prohibited RTÉ from conducting interviews with members of proscribed organisations such as the IRA. That meant that people in RTÉ were extremely paranoid about all on-screen appearances, especially live interviews. If you spoke up against Section 31 – known as 'the ban' – on the grounds that, say, denying a voice to extremists may ultimately prove counterproductive and instead serve to prolong the conflict in the North, you ran the risk of being branded a Provo sympathiser. Many people didn't speak up because they didn't want the hassle of being branded. Few broadcasters agreed with the directive or thought that it contributed in any meaningful way to a peaceful resolution of the Northern Troubles. However, it was a government order and so everyone was stuck with it.

Most of the time, 'the ban' played no part in my working life. The only time that Section 31 became a factor in my work on the *Late Late* was when I was assigned to research a debate on Northern Ireland between the Northern priest Fr Dennis Faul and the politician who was responsible for Section 31, Conor Cruise O'Brien. A crucial aspect was to ensure that no Provos or members of other paramilitary organisations snuck into the audience to participate in the live debate.

The only other occasion when Section 31 had a direct impact on me was when I went for an interview for a radio producer job on 2fm. Someone on the panel asked me for my thoughts on Section 31. I was hung over and I had arrived late to the interview and I completely blanked. I couldn't recall what Section 31 was all about. In my fuddled state, I mistook it for the controversial rule that insisted that Irish-made records should constitute a certain percentage of 2fm's pop music play list. That rule meant lots of exposure for crap show bands as well as second-rate country-and-Irish singers.

'Well, I disagree with it,' I said confidently.

The three old guys on the panel gave me their full attention.

'We're giving far too much exposure to show bands,' I continued.

The panel looked puzzled. Had the IRA subverted the country's show bands? Was Big Tom's massive hit 'Four Roads to Glenamady' a secret IRA code? Did I know something that they didn't?

After a few more questions, it became clear to them that I had no idea what I was talking about. The panel appeared deeply concerned that I didn't know about Section 31, as well they might, considering that I had been working in RTÉ for a year by then.

The interview died. For a time, we sat in silence and looked at each other like lizards on a rock.

I left the room feeling like a dork. Halfway along the corridor, I suddenly grasped the meaning of Section 31. I felt like running back into the room yelling 'I've remembered, I've remembered', but I doubt that the panel would have been impressed by that either.

I didn't get a second interview.

★

At the *Late Late*, I did my work and kept my head down. I suggested guests and topics, including quite a few panel discussions featuring the opinions of young people that could have been subtitled 'What are our young people of today really thinking?' or 'Meet the movers and shakers of the future'.

I convinced Muireann, a pal from college days, to appear on a *Late Late* panel to talk about being young and female in Ireland. Muireann had been sharing an apartment with two artist friends, both men. It was an innocent arrangement and I told Gay about it merely as background information.

On the night, Gay asked Muireann what it was like to live with two men. The question put her in an awkward spot and she struggled. Everything she said only seemed to reinforce the impression that she had chosen to sexually co-habit with two men. The interview was no longer about being young and female in Ireland, instead it addressed her perceived sex life.

Afterwards, Muireann was mortified. Her mother didn't even know about her accommodation arrangements. Now the whole country would think that she was a trollop. I felt remorse about that, but Gay shrugged it off as part of the deal. He said that I shouldn't have mentioned it in my briefing to him.

I recommended various bands to Howard, who booked the entertainment for the show and was keen to give a break to new and exciting acts. At my suggestion Howard gave The Virgin Prunes a gig. The Virgin Prunes were Ireland's only performance art rock band. They liked to dress in colourful costumes, including women's clothing. They used eyeliner and mascara and painted their faces and bodies weird colours. There was always an artistic point to their noisy, in-your-face performances, but usually only the band themselves knew it. Not noted for their musical ability or melodic songs, they baffled and frequently outraged audiences on their rare live appearances, but they were rarely dull. I wanted to see what effect they would have on a *Late Late* audience who were mainly used to a home-grown musical diet of Daddy Cool and the Lollipops, Brendan Shine and other show band or cabaret acts.

Gay didn't like most pop or rock music. He was usually scornful of rock bands, though he would never prevent a guest or an act or a band from appearing just because he didn't like them. If it was good for the *Late Late*, it got on.

'OK,' Gay said when we put it to him at the Tuesday meeting. 'But they had better be good.'

On the following Saturday, the Prunes arrived, looking like a medieval circus troupe. The band did a quick camera rehearsal. After that they went to their dressing room and really dolled themselves up. At one stage Guggi roamed the corridor outside Studio One trying to locate a more outrageous-looking tie than the one he had brought with him. He even tried several from Gay's wardrobe before finally reverting to his original choice.

On air, the band looked like a bunch of pre-Raphaelite serial killers. They posed, tossed their heads, glared at the audience from scary, heavily mascaraed eye sockets, gesticulated and screamed out lyrics that nobody could understand. They made a lot of noise, and they were wonderful.

The Prunes' appearance on the show provoked a stream of angry phone calls. One phone call came through to the hospitality room. 'Can you explain to me what these pagans are doing on our TV screens?'

I told him that the Prunes were Ireland's first performance art rock band. The caller was unimpressed. 'Right, I'm taking this to a higher authority,' he said and hung up.

The Prunes were delighted by the response. Gavin, the lead singer, told me their intention was to provoke a reaction. Audience indifference would have constituted failure. In that respect, The Virgin Prunes had a lot in common with Gay Byrne.

Gay thought the music was terrible, but he enjoyed The Virgin Prunes' visual impact. 'I'm glad that they have a good stage image because they're going to need it,' he said.

U2 were best friends with the Prunes but they were a lot easier to sell. I had also recommended U2 for an appearance, although Howard said he was going to book them anyway because they were making quite a splash in the post-punk scene. They had been tipped as the next Irish band to make it after The Boomtown Rats.

A *Late Late* appearance could be intimidating. Bands used to the buzz and excitement of a gig in a rock venue found themselves gazing out at the bland, indifferent faces of a middle-age, middle-brow *Late Late* audience that often looked like they had wandered in for a bingo night.

U2 were nervous, but they went down well. They seemed young in person, but on camera they looked like schoolboys. However, the music and performance were polished and mature – though nobody reckoned that they were destined to become the next Rats.

Afterwards over drinks in the hospitality room, U2 were polite and respectful and interested in the opinions of others. Bono and The Edge were excellent conversationalists. Squeezed into undersized rickety chairs, they debated issues of the day with the conservative radio and newspaper agony aunt, Angela McNamara. At the end of the night the rock band and the agony aunt swapped phone numbers. U2 came across as four talented and deeply committed but genuinely nice and unpretentious guys. They were in complete contrast to the traditional rock-band image of a bunch of doomed, narcissistic, leather-jacketed cynics who had just stepped out of the cult movie, *The Wild One*. U2 were more boy scouts than bikers, but they weren't phonies. At the postmortem, Gay described U2 as 'lovely lads'.

★

One day a disagreement arose between Gay and Howard. On Saturday night some band had turned up with an instrumental and vocal line-up that was allegedly different to the one supplied by Howard at the Tuesday meeting. The mix-up had caused delay and confusion. Howard disputed Gay's version of events. Gay insisted on getting to the bottom of the problem. Things got heated. Howard was a dignified man with a glorious, deeply resonant voice, like the *Late Late*'s answer to Richard Burton. He stood up and informed Gay in sonorous tones that he had had enough of Gay's nonsense. Howard then walked out, slamming the door behind him.

Everyone remained silent as we watched Howard walk across the tarmac to his own annex opposite. We saw him open the door and disappear inside. We heard his footsteps tramping across the floor to his desk by the window. We watched as he sat down at his desk.

Gay waited patiently until Howard was seated at his desk before picking up his phone and dialling. Everyone pretended to be deeply involved in their work. In the distance, we heard a phone ringing. We watched Howard answer his phone. 'Don't you ever fucking slam the door on me again,' Gay said sternly.

Then he slammed down the phone.

Across the way, Howard also slammed down his receiver and then he rose from his desk and disappeared. A few moments later, he reappeared outside his annex, marching purposefully towards the *Late Late* office.

Even the chairs in the *Late Late* office tensed as Howard disappeared around the corner. Gay remained calm, studying some paperwork.

There was a moment's silence before the door to the *Late Late* office burst open. Howard stood in the doorway glaring fiercely at Gay. 'And don't you ever fucking slam the phone down on me again,' he roared, and then he slammed the door behind him. Gay continued to study the papers on his desk.

This time Howard walked across the tarmac and passed by his own annex to vanish around the corner.

Afterwards at the coffee break, the rest of the team agreed that it had been a cracking row, one of the best of the season. Apparently, really vicious rows were rare in the *Late Late*, which was essentially a happy, hard-working and highly motivated team. However, Gay and Howard were good for a couple of good jousts per season. They had worked together for a long while and got along well most of the time, but they had built up a bit of history. They each liked to let off steam, often while the other was in the firing line.

★

The only time I saw Gay Byrne rattled about an item was at the prospect of an interview with the black American writer James Baldwin. Gay wasn't too comfortable with literary heavyweights, and the prospect of coaxing a good relevant interview out of a black, homosexual, intellectual novelist and essayist who was deeply devoted to issues of race and gender equality may possibly have represented Gay's worst night-mare. Gay's main issue was that he wasn't sure if Baldwin would make good television. People had heard of Baldwin, but they just hadn't heard *from* him for a long while. Nevertheless, Baldwin was one of the great writers of our times and was worth having on the show.

Gay enjoyed interviewing the successful thriller writer and excellent raconteur Frederick Forsyth. Forsyth's good-humoured, erudite and engaging storytelling had made him a *Late Late* regular, along with Gay's other favourites Peter Ustinov and Billy Connolly.

I went to meet Baldwin at the Gresham Hotel a day before the show. He was surrounded by burly black minders, one of whom interviewed me for twenty minutes before allowing me anywhere near the man himself. I wasn't an expert on Baldwin's work. However, I had read and loved *Go Tell It on the Mountain* and *Giovanni's Room* along with the short-story col-lection, *Going to Meet the Man*. I was able to answer all of the questions that the minder asked. Once he realised that I wasn't a complete chancer, he appeared relieved and became friendly. He didn't want Baldwin getting stitched up on live TV, he told me. They had had some torrid experiences in the US.

Baldwin was a tiny man in his late fifties who moved like a

ballet dancer. He had an enormous face with large, protruding eyes that could make him appear either fierce or frightened. He seemed to relax only when he was talking. He had a powerful presence made even more extraordinary by his resonant, hypnotic voice. Once he started speaking, he didn't stop. I was enraptured by that rich voice, even though there were times when he drifted into a lyrical but impenetrable reverie.

On the night, I went to Gay's dressing room to give him some last-minute notes. Gay rarely took written notes; he relied on his memory and never forgot an important piece of information and he absolutely never neglected to ask the question that the viewer at home wanted to ask. The problem with Baldwin was that he wasn't sure what the viewer at home might want to know.

Gay appeared as relaxed as usual. He stared at himself in the mirror as he often did before a show, psyching himself up in a typically self-contained way. 'OK, son, go ahead,' he said softly. 'Tell me about Baldwin.'

I gave Gay some final details. Then I suggested that he ask Baldwin if he thought that conditions for black people in America had changed much since he started writing. 'As long as he's a good talker,' Gay said.

Gay gave Baldwin a rousing introduction and welcomed him to *The Late Late Show*. Then Gay asked a question and Baldwin took off. He spoke for nearly twenty minutes. Gay looked like he was travelling in the passenger seat of a car that had lost its driver.

After a few minutes nobody was entirely certain what Baldwin was talking about, but his voice and his presence were spellbinding. Baldwin was a fast-flowing river and to attempt to interrupt him was to jump in and risk being carried away. Best to let the river go where it may. Gay wisely stayed quiet.

However when Baldwin finished, the audience gave him warm and generous applause. Perhaps they were relieved that

an unusual and sometimes mystifying monologue had finished, but there were genuine feelings of affection as well as
admiration for Baldwin. They liked his passionate intelligence.

A week later I got a thank-you note from the burly minder.
The note was addressed to 'Ferdia Mac Banana, Late Late
Show, RTÉ'.

★

One Saturday night I was delegated to help Ces to look after
Oliver Reed. Ces was with Reed at the actor's hotel. She had
phoned the office to say that he was drinking half pints of
whiskey and was insisting that she match him drink for drink.
She could use a little help.

Somehow, Ces managed to get Reed back to the *Late Late*
hospitality room just before the show was due to start. I was
standing by the drinks table smoking a cigarette when Reed
came in. The first thing he did was lean forward to bite the end
off my lit cigarette. He made a big deal of chewing and swal-
lowing and then he patted his stomach, twirling the end of an
invisible moustache like an English aristocrat who had just
risen from a delicious feast. 'Aaaaah,' he said. 'By Jove.'

Reed's wife arrived. She remained selflessly in the corner as
he went about the room, introducing himself to people and
generally messing about. Then he came back to the drinks
table to politely request a large whiskey. One moment he was
chatting to me about the beauties of rural Ireland, the next he
was attempting to balance upside down on a chair using one
arm. He had seen Keith Moon do it, he said (The Who was his
favourite band). Reed fell off the chair and sprawled on the
floor of the hospitality room.

There was no talk of not allowing Reed to appear, despite the
fact that the show was going out live and that he had clearly been
drinking a lot. On screen, Gay was interviewing Susan George.

Reed stared up at the hospitality TV. 'I like Susan,' he announced suddenly. 'I think I'm going to throw her over the sofa.'

But when the time came for Reed to go on, he suddenly ran off. Gay's announcement of 'Ladies and gentlemen – Oliver Reed' was met by a round of applause but no sign of Reed. After a few breathless moments of dead air, Maura discovered Reed hiding behind the stage curtains like a mischievous schoolboy. She led the giggling actor to the side of the set and the floor manager brought him on.

After that, Reed went wild.

One of the first things he did was to keep his promise to throw Susan George over the sofa. Next he tried to balance on a chair using one hand again. This time he succeeded, gaining a warm round of applause. Everyone was mesmerised by his drunken antics. It didn't matter that the interview fell apart within seconds or that Reed was obviously completely out of his tree, it still made riveting television.

In hospitality I stood alongside Reed's wife throughout. From time to time she gave a small shrill laugh. 'Oh that was funny, Oliver,' she said to the television screen above her.

The phone lines lit up with viewers complaining, a sure sign that the show was a big ratings success.

Afterwards Gay decided to go to a nightclub with the team, the only time during my two seasons with the show that he went on the town. Gay's version of partying was to enjoy a couple of drinks, engage in long, boisterous chats with colleagues and occasional souls who wandered over to meet the TV legend and hit the floor for a brief dance before heading for home. That was the first time I really noticed that Gay rarely seemed to carry either money or cigarettes – he usually smoked other people's.

The postmortem the following Tuesday was a congratulatory affair, a celebration of a show that the whole country was still talking about and that had made number one. Audience ratings during Reed's appearance had gone off the scale.

Reed had phoned someone on the team at the weekend expressing deep remorse. He felt that he had not given a true account of himself and begged to be allowed to appear this coming Saturday to redress the balance. Someone suggested that it would be good to have Reed back as long as he was sober. The suggestion was approved. Reed returned to the show the following Saturday. He was sober, easy-going, friendly and full of stories about his acting life.

He was a total bore.

Viewers liked Oliver Reed as a drunken loon. They weren't interested in watching him give a 'true account' of himself.

★

On Thursday nights I often went to the Rockabilly Record Hop in the Magnet bar on Pearse Street. The Hops were held upstairs in a big function room and drew a large crowd of Teds, young rockabillies, bikers, Hell's Angels and music fans. The DJ was Stompin' George, a big man who often wore a long leather trench coat that made him look like a hitman in a French movie. Rockin' Kevin, a real life Teddy Boy who had first put on drapes in the Dublin of the late fifties, handled meet-and-greet duties at the door. Kevin always wore his finest Teddy Boy drapes and brothel creepers.

It was a lively scene, packed with colourful characters as well as lots of people who didn't belong to a gang or genre but simply adored the music. Despite the potential combustibility of the patrons, there was never any trouble at the Rockabilly Hops. Road rockers mixed with young Teds and rockabillies got along fine with Hell's Angels and punks.

I was still interested in getting a Hell's Angel on the *Late Late*. I talked to Mac, the leader of the Irish chapter of the Hell's Angels. Mac was a quiet-spoken Englishman who led a group of about half-a-dozen Angels, along with around a dozen or so 'prospects' or apprentices who had yet to earn their 'colours', the leather jacket with the official Angels' logo that a fully fledged member always wore and never washed. Mac was willing to go on the *Late Late* to talk about life as an Angel in Ireland and abroad, but he wanted one hundred pounds in cash. As Mac saw things, if he appeared on the *Late Late* he was handing Gay Byrne carte blanche to make a fool out of him. Mac had no problem with that – that was Gay's job – but he reckoned that one hundred quid would be adequate compensation for the humiliation.

I put it to Gay – and Gay said no. 'I get Freddie Forsyth for the usual fee. Why should I pay a hundred pounds for an Irish Hell's Angel who isn't even Irish?'

At the Magnet, I heard about a legendary Welsh Teddy Boy and rock-and-roll record collector, Breathless Dan Coffey. He now lived in Fermanagh with his blonde girlfriend, Frantic Fay. I felt strongly that Dan had the potential to make an interesting and very different guest for the *Late Late*, if he could be persuaded to appear.

I pitched the notion to Gay and he told me to go up to Fermanagh to meet with Dan. 'Find out if he can talk,' Gay told me. 'He may be the reincarnation of Elvis, but he's of no use to me if he can't put two words together.'

I convinced Howard to drive me up. We invited Rockin Kevin along as our inside man. Kevin was over six feet tall and easy-going. He wore his hair with a quiff. He was a friendly guy, who loved music but he didn't strike me as a man to be messed with, he was a tough guy.

Dan could be a bit difficult, it appeared. Having Rockin Kevin along would put him at ease. At least, so we thought.

We had just driven over the border when I discovered that back in the early sixties Dan had taken offence at something Kevin said or did and challenged him to a duel. The invitation had been accepted, but circumstances as well as the passing of years had prevented it from occurring.

Now I was rattled. Did that mean that Kevin and Dan were likely to fight a duel some time during our visit to Fermanagh? 'Aw, no,' Kevin said. 'Sure I've seen him a good few times since and he's never mentioned it. He's probably forgotten all about it.'

Kevin sat up in his seat and adjusted his cuffs. 'Course if he hasn't, well, I'm always ready…'

I spent the rest of the journey wondering what I might have gotten myself into.

Dan lived in a fine house in a remote part of the Fermanagh countryside. He wore a stylish black frock coat and string tie. He looked like a landed gentleman from the American Deep South.

Inside, a Confederate flag hung on his wall next to a Tricolour. Dan was a sturdy man with penetrating eyes. He was cordial and he laughed easily, but it was like being in the company of a caged tiger. The man was primed, ready to explode. He seemed to be containing a lot of rage that had built up over the years. He reminded me of a Welsh version of the rock legend and unpredictable fireball Jerry Lee Lewis. Despite his gentlemanly manners, Dan made you feel that he would not hesitate to pull a pistol on you to avenge a perceived slight. I liked him, but he was intimidating.

He brought us into his music room, which had an old Pye record player and a pair of colossal speakers in the centre. The walls were lined with shelves of vinyl records, all meticulously arranged. He boasted that he could lay his hands in seconds on virtually any old rock-and-roll record I could name. He dared me to ask for something obscure. He was testing me.

I knew a lot about rockabilly at this stage. I had spent a lot of time in the house of a friend of mine called Billy ('Boppin Billy' whenever he DJ-ed), who had a massive collection of all kinds of music and who had turned me on to quite a few rock-abilly legends such as Johnny Burnette and Warren Smith, not to mention minor players such as Hardrock Gunther, Billy 'Crash' Craddock and H-Bomb Ferguson.

I asked Dan for anything by Eddie Bush (a guitarist who had played with minor rockabilly legend Carl Mann amongst others). Breathless Dan made a few moves and had a single by Eddie Bush out of its sleeve and carefully laid on the turntable within twenty seconds. 'I've only played this a couple of times,' he said. 'It's quite rare.'

He produced a box of needles for the Pye record player. The needles were large, jagged spikes. He told us that as far as he knew, the box contained the last remaining batch of needles for this particular model. He wasn't sure what he was going to do when they ran out. He found himself cutting back on his disc spinning time just to preserve the needles and that was not a good thing.

Frantic Fay was blonde and could have stepped straight out of the movie *American Graffiti*. She wore a colourful top and springy fifties dress. Her glasses were slim cat's eyes. She didn't have much to say, preferring to leave the talking to Dan. They had been world rock-and-roll dance champions but they rarely did exhibitions nowadays, they had picked up niggling injuries. The venues were never as good as the old days.

We spent about three hours with Dan. He came across as a complex character, polite one moment, prickly the next. It was hard to relax in his company.

Dan was very big on honour. He showed us a newsletter he had written where he had challenged a man to a duel with guns or knives. The man had offended Dan and Dan was not prepared to let that go. He was coy on whether the duel had ever taken place. I got the impression that the man had left town, but that Dan had kept the invitation open. He wanted us to know that he had once done business this way, and would not be averse to doing so again should the need arise.

I kept expecting him to produce a pair of duelling pistols and ask me to be his second in the duel with Kevin. Instead,

Dan and Kevin showed enormous respect for each other. Neither seemed keen to get into a situation where they might clash. In a confrontation between the two rockers, it was obvious that neither man would give an inch.

Dan was ambivalent about the *Late Late*. He often watched the show. He didn't think he would get along with the host. He didn't know if he could dance anymore because of injury, and it would be hard to know what he was going to talk about if he couldn't dance or play rock-and-roll records. He said he'd have a big think about an appearance.

We said goodbye and left Dan and Fay in their Deep South time capsule.

On the drive home I struggled with the notion of putting Dan on the *Late Late*. In the end, I decided against it. Dan was essentially a quiet man. He represented a love of fifties rock and roll that was coupled with a way of life that had almost vanished. He was a fifties throwback. I decide that he would be an excellent subject for a TV documentary, but I figured that he would be lost on the *Late Late*.

However, there was something else bothering me about Dan and I couldn't work out what it was.

The next morning I told Gay of my impressions about Dan. I told him that I didn't feel that he would be a good interview at this time.

Gay listened to what I had to say and then he looked at me. 'You think he's vulnerable, don't you?'

I thought for a moment. He was right. I was worried about what might happen during Dan's appearance on live TV. I didn't trust Gay. I thought about what had happened with my friend Muireann. After that, I had sworn that I would take more care with the people I recommended to appear. I sensed that something bad would happen if Dan went on the show.

'Yes,' I said. 'He won't be a good guest.'

'Good,' Gay said. 'Well done. You made the right decision.'

★

An RTÉ producer named John McColgan joined the *Late Late* team for a few weeks. He had produced a special on the songs of singer-songwriter Dory Previn, who had just published her autobiography. McColgan suggested that Dory would make a good guest for the show. Gay agreed.

Untypically, Gay agreed to have dinner with Dory the night before the show, something he had never done before. Gay liked to meet the guests on air so that the interaction was fresh.

During the interview, Dory said that she would talk about anything as long as Gay didn't ask about her abortion. The subject was still too close and she was simply too vulnerable to deal with it. Apparently Gay agreed not to mention it.

On the night of the interview, one of Gay's first questions was to ask Dory about her abortion. Dory freaked. Gay kept on probing as sensitively as he could, but the damage was done. Dory wouldn't answer. She mentioned that Gay had promised not to ask her about the abortion. She said that she couldn't believe he was going back on his word. Gay kept going, and the interview stuttered and stopped but it didn't grind to a halt. Dory didn't walk off. The discomfort and friction between interviewer and guest made absorbing television, but we were all shocked that Gay had reneged on his promise.

Afterwards there was anger and disillusionment. In the dressing room, some of the team remonstrated with Gay about changing his mind on asking the abortion question.

Gay appeared defiant. 'Watch the ratings,' he said. He was right – they soared during the Dory Previn interview and the show made number one again.

The portmortem was dominated by the Dory Previn abortion question as well as by discussion of Gay's broken promise. Someone made the point that the *Late Late* ran on trust. How could any of us trust him now?

Gay took us all on. He made the point that Dory had written about the abortion in her autobiography, so the issue was in the public domain. He had asked a legitimate and relevant question. He would not have been doing his job if he had stuck to his agreement. Gay would have looked stupid to the viewers at home if he had not asked her about it, because that was the question that the viewers would want to ask her. He conceded that it might have been a mistake to go to dinner with Dory on the Friday, but once she appeared on his show she was fair game.

McColgan said that he was disappointed. Apparently, Dory Previn was still broken up about things. There was no resolution and the meeting eventually moved on to the following Saturday's show without much enthusiasm.

The next morning, it emerged that Gay had apologised to McColgan. That pissed off some of the team. At the Friday meeting, I asked why he had not apologised to us as well. We were the ones who worked with him week by week. We needed to feel that we could trust him. But Gay didn't feel he had to apologise to us. As far as he was concerned, the item and the show had been a success. Once a celebrity (or anyone, for that matter) agreed to be interviewed on the *Late Late*, they belonged to him while they were on air. The celebrity was selling something, and they had no right to complain about the questions they were asked. Gay had given us a hard lesson in the reality of live TV. He had been number one for a long time, and he intended to remain at the top of his profession for as long as he could. We had been given a reality check on what made him – as well as the show – successful.

An unwritten rule emerged in the wake of the Dory Previn business. If you didn't want Gay to ask about something, you didn't mention it to him.

★

One night after a show, Gay gave me a lift home. As we were stopped at a traffic light, a red van pulled up alongside. There were two men in the van and they looked across at Gay with interest. Gay had his window rolled down. The guy in the passenger seat of the red van seemed deep in thought. He rolled down his window and leaned out.

'Hey,' he said.

'Hello there,' Gay said cheerfully.

'You know,' the man said smugly, 'If I'd a face like yours, I'd look like Gay Byrne.'

Just then the lights changed and the red van roared off. We heard raucous laughter drifting back to us.

'They are all out there,' Gay said. 'All kinds of people.'

★

I left *The Late Late Show* at the end of my second season.

I wanted to move on and do something else. I liked working on the *Late Late*, but I didn't want to stay as a researcher. I was restless. I wanted to find something that I really loved to do. Besides, the prospect of a job as a radio producer had disappeared.

Gay didn't like people leaving his team, which was like a family. At the season-wrap party he wished me well, but he told me that I was making a mistake.

I didn't think I would miss the *Late Late*, but I did. Most of the other programmes that I worked on after it were colourless or lame in comparison.

14

Beer and Blood and Rockandroll

Everyone said I was mad to quit my job in RTÉ to go on the road with a new band, The Rhythm Kings. I knew that they were right and sensible, but I couldn't help myself. I was going nowhere in RTÉ. I'd miss the live excitement of the *Late Late* where anything could happen, but I didn't want to feel trapped as a TV researcher for the rest of my days.

I was twenty-four and antsy again. I wanted to do something big before I grew too old. I could feel my bones fossilising by the hour in RTÉ. I was losing confidence. It felt as though my life had ended. My old shyness returned. I remembered only the good experiences from my time in the Gravediggers. In a band, every night felt like Saturday night. In RTÉ, every morning felt like a Monday.

Besides, I had unfinished business with rock and roll. I had never recorded and released either a single or an album. The Gravediggers had vanished without leaving a legacy, except some demo and live tapes as well as a rockabilly ditty (from our unreleased recordings for Good Vibrations) that had ended up on *Just For Kicks* (a compilation album of new Irish rock that also featured tracks from The Teen Commandments, The New Versions and U2). I wanted to show that I was more than just a controversial stage name. I wanted to become an Irish rock star. I wanted an excuse to wear sunglasses indoors and I wanted an easy way to meet girls. Most of all, I wanted to write songs and release an album that I could be proud of.

In the early eighties, Ireland was a land of grey skies and greyer people. The country suffered from massive unemployment and a huge emigration drain. The Troubles in the North seemed to be never-ending and unsolvable. Like a lot of people in the South, most of the time I pretended that the North didn't exist. A heroin epidemic raged in Dublin, spreading into most of the major cities in the South. Every couple of months there was a bus strike or a bin strike or another form of industrial unrest. People clung to permanent pensionable jobs as though clutching to life rafts. Yet, to me, it seemed like a perfect time to start another rock band.

I still talked about writing a novel, but I didn't have the patience or the inspiration. There were too many things in my head. I wasn't ready yet. I wrote rock reviews and features for *In Dublin* magazine, *Hot Press* and *The Sunday Independent*, but that just made things worse. In January 1980 I interviewed U2 for *In Dublin*, the band's first cover story. They were making a noise in London and they said that things were much better organised over there. In Dublin, even brilliant bands suffered due to a lack of direction. 'Look at it this way,' Bono said. 'If you're a fifty-pence piece in a pile of ten-pence pieces you have to shine that much brighter in order to be noticed.'

I figured that being in a full-time band would cure me of my restlessness. Maybe it would give me something to write about. I decided to keep a diary – that way I could cover all the bases.

In the Gravediggers I had been immature. It was my first band and I'd known zilch about the music business. This time I knew what I was doing. I felt I could be a 'shiny fifty-pence piece', no problem.

As an example of my new maturity, I wrote a letter of resignation to RTÉ and then I invested in a PA system with my friend and rhythm guitarist, Ritchie.

I swam away from the RTÉ life raft as fast as I could. And it felt good.

Ritchie and I wrote a batch of songs. We brought back The Lizard on guitar and recruited Clint on bass. Clint was a tall, eccentric post-grad in archaeology who always wore the air of an aristocrat who had somehow ended up playing bass in a rock band. We found a drummer and saxophonist. We rehearsed for months in a dusty room in a dilapidated building on Dorset Street that belonged to The Individual, our saxophonist.

I worried more about keeping the stage name of Rocky De Valera than about a regular income. Finally, I decided that there was no way that I could ever lose it, unless I could think of an even wilder, more irreverent name. Lots of people still called me Rocky. Even my girlfriend Jenny said it made sense to retain Rocky.

I wanted the new group to take its inspiration and musical style from a Texas blues band, The Fabulous Thunderbirds, who I'd seen in London sometime in 1980. The Thunderbirds had worn sharp jackets and Hawaiian shirts. They looked cool and they played laid-back modern Texas blues. I thought they were the best band I had ever seen.

The Rhythm Kings would become the first Irish band to hit the big time by looking cool and playing modern blues with a bit of swagger.

We had no real competition. Dublin was a fashion disaster. Punk style had disappeared, though there were still several hardcore mohicans around Grafton Street. Instead, hundreds of New Romantic mullet-headed fops roamed the streets, looking as though they had failed auditions for Duran Duran. All the women in nightclubs looked like Boy George.

Somebody had to provide an antidote.

Ritchie and I couldn't find Hawaiian shirts anywhere in Dublin. Instead we bought black shirts and white slim-Jim ties and zoot suits in Hairy Legs. I found a pair of two-tone brothel creepers. The Lizard said we looked like Dublin's answer to the Kray twins, but I thought we looked the business.

We composed a three-part plan for success.

First: build up a following.

Second: record and release hit singles and an album.

Third: move to London.

Simple. We couldn't fail – as long as we stuck to the plan.

For the first year we played as many gigs as we could hustle all over the country. We built up a following, gaining a reputation as a good, sweaty live band. It went to our heads.

We gave a better stage show than The Bogey Boys. We wrote better songs than The Atrix. We dressed cooler than Tokyo Olympics. We thought we were sharper looking than The Lookalikes.

Our first single, 'Goin' Steady', came in a dark sleeve with our picture on the front. We didn't look like The Fabulous Thunderbirds, but we thought we looked cool, even though the photograph had been taken in the graveyard of a local church.

En route to the Macroom Festival, we heard ourselves on the radio for the first time. Immediately, we screamed at Sigmund Freud, our driver, to pull the van into the side of the road. We listened to 'Goin' Steady' until it faded. I felt great pride along with a sense of joy that made me feel as though I was floating. Then the DJ praised the record as a terrific debut from a new Dublin band, 'The Rhythm Stars'. My good feelings fizzled away like air from a child's balloon.

That was my first inkling that success would not be an easy

or uncomplicated process. I suspected that I might have been deluding myself again.

But I got over it when we played an early evening slot at the Macroom Festival and went down well. Afterwards in the beer tent, people said we were going to 'go international'. We watched famous people get drunk and fall over. A girl made a pass at The Lizard. We got invited to parties. After an hour in the beer tent, we were the best rock band on the planet.

After midnight, our manager Dangerous Abe Cohen rounded everyone up and piled us into the van to head for Clonakilty to Noel Redding's house, where we were staying. Noel had played bass with Jimi Hendrix, but now he played gigs around Cork with his partner Carol, an attractive American who wore tinted glasses. They ran a rehearsal-room-cum-guesthouse for bands.

We got hopelessly lost on narrow winding roads in the dark. The Individual was positive that he knew the way and kept giving 'advice' and 'directions' for short cuts. We got to the point where if anyone recommended that we go one way, Sigmund Freud immediately turned the van around and shot off in the opposite direction.

Eventually, we arrived at Redding's house around three in the morning. He was waiting for us with tea, bread and butter and loads of Jimi Hendrix anecdotes. Redding looked like he had just stepped off the cover of Sgt Pepper, with psychedelic shades, masses of curly hair and a colourful eighteenth-century military jacket. His large, sparsely furnished house was set on an acre of rambling bumpy land. Redding had been there and done everything in rock and roll. He personified a way of life that most of us in the band had shaken hands with but did not know.

'Eat up chaps,' Redding said. 'The fridge is empty. I know too much about what happens to food when there's a rock band staying over.'

We sat up for hours, talking about music and bands and girls and the meaning of life as we knew it as sparks exploded out of the massive fireplace and into our teacups. A strange sixties mushroom-shaped lampshade hung from the ceiling, throwing weird, flickering light onto the record collection that was propped against the wall, illuminating the face of Johnny Kidd, Gene Vincent, Joe Cocker and Jimi Hendrix as well as a young, psychedelic-shaded, massively afroed Noel Redding.

Redding put on *Johnny Kidd and the Pirates' Greatest Hits*. He placed the needle at the start of 'Shakin' All Over'. 'Do you hear that guitar lick?' he asked. 'I used to play that when I played lead. I taught his guitarist how to do it. Look, I'll show you.' He then demonstrated how to play the famous lick on an invisible guitar.

He said he'd heard a lot about our band and that he'd heard we were good. He told me that the important thing was to keep going, no matter what. Give it your best shot until you either made it or fell out with everyone. Then walk away and try to do something else. 'Only it's difficult to do something else,' he said quietly. 'Once the music gets into you, then that's usually that.'

★

After midnight one night, The Individual phoned to tell me that his house in Dorset Street had been broken into and our equipment had been stolen. The burglars had taken Lizard's guitar, Ritchie's guitar and The Individual's sax as well as his record player, speakers and record collection.

He had tracked the burglars to a block of flats across the street. By the time I arrived at three am, the balconies of the flats were lined with people. The night rang with catcalls and insults as the residents slagged off the policemen who were searching for our gear.

Eventually, a chap who claimed to be a social worker turned

up, offering to help. He knew some of these people; leave it to him and he would see what could be done. The 'social worker' disappeared into the flats, returning a while later with an offer from the burglars. We could have the gear back for three hundred quid. 'The kids who have taken your gear think you're rich because you're in a band,' he said.

The Individual scraped up a hundred and fifty. The rest of us contributed what we had on us, making a total of around two hundred.

'I think that will do it,' said the 'social worker'.

Just before The Individual handed over the money, a plain-clothes cop appeared. The cop was a small, stout man who walked everywhere in a hurry at a forward tilt. 'Before you get into that sort of thing, I'm just going to have another look around.' The plain-clothes cop summoned a couple of gardaí and went into the flats complex, vanishing into one of the alleyways. A few moments later, he emerged carrying a guitar. The two gardaí followed, carting the rest of our instruments.

The 'social worker' abruptly vanished. From the balconies above came a stream of curses and shouts and boos. Now every light in the block of flats seemed to be blazing. It looked like a scene from a Fellini movie. 'I found these at the bottom of a rubbish chute,' the plain-clothes cop said. 'I just had a hunch.'

★

A few months later we were booked to play The Olympia as support to Joe Jackson, who had become a big star. Joe met us for drinks beforehand. He hadn't changed much, except that he was a bit wary of being mobbed by fans and well-wishers. He snuck into the pub wearing a Gnarly Old Man mask. He still liked to wear white shoes, similar to the ones from the famous cover of his debut album, *Look Sharp*. He agreed to play piano with us during our gig. He would come on wearing the mask. We gave him a stage name, Paddy Kool. It would be a laugh.

On the way back to The Olympia Joe wore the Old Man mask again, but his white shoes gave him away. He was instantly recognised by the queues of people waiting to get into the gig. As our entourage passed by, the crowd sang 'Is She Really Going Out With Him'. Joe was touched. 'They sang it in tune,' he said. 'Well, almost.'

We played a strong, energetic set, and just before the last number introduced our special guest star, Paddy Kool. Joe came on in the mask and fooled nobody. He played piano on the last couple of numbers.

The Joe Jackson Band then played a storming set. It was one of the best nights I had ever experienced in music. I felt as though I knew what I was doing. I had made the right decision to leave my secure job in search of rock stardom.

We played Joe our demo tape. He liked it. We asked him if he would produce our album. He said we didn't need him. We already had a sound. We just needed a really good engineer and more strong songs.

Afterwards we went back to the bar in the lobby of Joe's hotel for drinks. The lobby was packed with conventioneers who had just piled out from a big boozy dinner. Everywhere you looked men in suits sang tuneless ballads, attempted to paw the waitresses or got into arguments, sometimes having to be pulled apart. At the front entrance, one suit helped another suit get sick into a potted plant while the porters looked on. Conventioneers sprawled across comfortable chairs, unconscious and snoring or with their mouths open. The hotel duty manager was not keen to let us have a drink in the lobby – it was too late and not all of us were residents. We tried to talk him into it, but he told us that we would have to leave and get a late-night drink elsewhere.

The duty manager escorted us to the door in case we got up to rock band mischief on our way out. The Rhythm Kings and the Joe Jackson Band walked quietly out of the hotel while all around us conventionally attired, middle-aged, middle-class men in suits fell about like skittles being tumbled by invisible bowling balls.

★

On the way to a gig in Cavan, every pole we passed had a black flag billowing from it as marks of respect to the H-Block hunger strikers who were engaged in a political protest to the death in the Maze Prison. The flags had appeared several miles outside Dublin, and the further we got from the capital, the more of them appeared. They hung from telegraph poles and postboxes. They flapped from streetlights as we drove through small towns. Black flags fluttered from the wing mirrors of cars we passed.

Around thirty miles from King's Court, the accelerator cable in our Volkswagen van snapped. Our new driver, Bozo, improvised a temporary brake cable utilising one of Clint's bass guitar strings. Attaching the bass string to the broken accelerator cable at the back of the van, Bozo then tied it to a tow rope that he carefully threaded through a hole in the rear window, over the amplifiers and drums and guitars and past our seats to the passenger seat and into the hands of our drummer, Wong. On Bozo's command – 'Poke, Wong, poke' – the drummer pulled on the cable and off we stuttered. The temporary arrangement got us to a large hall in the middle of King's Court, Cavan.

We entered a magnificently ornate ballroom complete with a carpeted stage. We set up the gear for a sound check while Bozo drove off to find a mechanic, steering with one hand while his free hand tugged on the tow rope.

Everyone hated the ballroom gigs. They were not rock gigs

and there was no way to justify them to ourselves. We did them for the money and that was all. Occasionally, a ballroom gig metamorphosed into a rock-and-roll gig because of good audience reaction, but that was a rarity. Most of the time audiences in ballrooms were so steeped in the show-band, country-and-western tradition that they stood about waiting for us to play a country number so they could dance. We didn't play country numbers. That meant that most of the time the audiences stood looking at us with blank faces. There was rarely any applause. Some nights the audience response was so vacant that it felt as though we had wandered onto a remake of *Night of the Living Dead.*

Only about eighty 'living dead' showed up for this gig. A third of them turned out to be ardent H-Block patriots. One had a T-shirt with Bobby Sands' face emblazoned on it.

At the end of the night we walked off stage without playing the national anthem. We were a rock band. We didn't play national anthems.

The crowd ranted and stomped their feet and shouted. They hammered on the dressing-room door. We thought that they wanted an encore – they had loved us after all.

Then Bozo came in pale faced to tell us that the H-Blockers were about to trash our gear because they had taken grave offence at our refusal to play the anthem.

The noise outside became a cacophony. Bozo ducked out for a look and quickly returned, urging us to prepare for an attack. We heard thumping and kicking outside our dressing room. The door rocked on its hinges.

Ritchie and Lizard grabbed their guitars and held them over their shoulders like baseball bats. The only weapon I could find was a small empty Fanta bottle.

Suddenly the door burst open. A mass of red, angry faces appeared, pushing and shoving and holding each other back in the doorway. 'Whywontyisplaythefugginanthem?' one guy yelled.

I explained as calmly as I could that we were a rock band and we didn't play anthems. We should play the anthem, they yelled. It was an insult to Irishmen that we didn't play it. Was it because we were from Dublin? Were we Brits or what?

I argued that they wouldn't expect Thin Lizzy or Bruce Springsteen to play the national anthem after a gig. There was a brief pause. 'Those people played the anthem when they were here,' yelled one red-faced thug.

We exited through the side door onto the stage, anxious to save our gear from getting trashed. Clint, still wearing his stage attire of blind-man's shades and white dinner jacket, stood calmly at the side of the stage looking unconcerned at the mayhem. The promoters tried desperately to calm the crowd down, but things got worse. Wong tried to prevent two of the toughest-looking H-Blockers from dismantling his drums. Others began climbing onto the stage to get at us.

Just as it looked like there was going to be a brawl, a soft voice suddenly began to sing the national anthem. We turned to find Clint singing into a microphone. The PA was still on so Clint's voice filled the hall. Soon it was joined by dozens of other voices as the H-Blockers sang along. Ritchie, The Individual, Wong and Lizard and I joined in.

When the singing was over, the same fanatics who had been about to lynch us cheered and shook our hands, congratulating us on a brilliant gig. We were the best band to play Cavan for years, they told us. They asked us for signed photographs and posters.

Afterwards, when the crowd had left the hall and the promoters had paid us, I told Clint that we had been extremely lucky.

Clint removed his blind-man shades and his eyes twinkled. 'Nonsense, we were never in any danger,' he said.

While we were loading the van, the local skinheads came up to apologise for the behaviour of the crowd.

★

Extract from Rocky's diary
Roundstone, 16 November 1981

The beautiful Stanley girls from Clifden and about fifty others were the only ones to show up for a gig that we had packed out during the summer. Wong was depressed. Ritchie angry. The Individual talked loudly, mainly to hear the sound of his own voice. The town itself was dark and menacing. The only hotel was closed down, taking away the focal point of the whole town. Strangers click-clacked through the cobbled streets, staring wildly at us at they passed, as though they were shocked to discover a rock band in their midst.

In the morning, all was different. The sun blazed. Huge splashes of light all over the town. The morning was bright but the wind was icy. I saw beautiful colours across the landscape. The eerie beauty of a blue-white speckled sky gave me a quiet joy. I noticed that the others had been affected as well. For a while we drove in silence, the sights stirring us. Then Bozo slapped on a tape and ruined the mood. The music was loud and distorted. It tore the stillness out of the morning.

We negotiated a deal to record and release 'John Wayne' on Scoff, an Irish record label. I was excited. This was more like it. Our second single should provide us with a breakthrough. I wasn't worried that I had written 'John Wayne' in ten minutes before a rehearsal, nor was I unduly concerned that the tune bore an uncanny similarity to the old fifties hit 'Wooly Bully' by Sam the Sham and the Pharoahs. It didn't even bother me that initially none of the band had wanted anything to do a song whose chorus ran: 'Is it a bird, is it a plane? No, no – it's John Wayne.' I finally convinced the others to include it in our set just for encores. As far as I was concerned, 'John Wayne' was in the tradition of rock-and-roll novelty records like 'Stranded in the Jungle' by The Cadets. I knew that it would give us a big hit.

We recorded the single in Lombard with Gerry Leonard producing. It was a difficult session, mainly because we had booked the studio from nine to five – fine for an ordinary day's work, but not for a rock band that had been gigging in Ballina the night before.

It didn't help when we spent an hour tuning up to the studio's grand piano only to discover that the piano was out of tune. We didn't get going until after lunch and we had to rush to finish in time.

A few weeks later I travelled to London with Dangerous Abe and BP Fallon, who had befriended us. BP set up meetings with seven record companies in two days. We were looking for a big album deal for the band. The least we hoped for was that an English record company would be impressed enough to give us a deal to release 'John Wayne' in the UK. Abe and I stayed in a large, rundown house belonging to a music journalist contact whose name we got from a friend. The house had a makeshift recording studio in the basement, at least two bands were sharing the upstairs bedrooms and there were cats everywhere. The morning we arrived a cat got run over on the road outside. Some of the guys in the house had a big funeral for it and buried it in the garden. They seemed really shaken. We slept downstairs on two sofas. The next morning, as we were leaving to meet the record companies, another cat got killed on the road.

Nobody was interested in 'John Wayne' or our demo tapes, except Stiff Records supremo Dave Robinson. He said that if we went back into the studio to record a decent version of 'Wayne', he would 'think about putting it out in the UK'. Our version was badly mixed, he said.

We got back to the house to find all the inhabitants deeply

upset because yet another cat had been creamed on the road. The music journalist was glad we were going back to Dublin. 'I'm not saying it's your fault,' he said, 'but all of those cats were alive before you guys arrived.'

When I got home, I talked to Ritchie about the situation. The whole London trip had been a waste of time. We shouldn't be going to see record companies. Record companies should be coming to see us. Dangerous Abe was not working out for us, we decided. He was too nice to be a manager. We didn't want to go back into the studio to re-record 'Wayne'. Instead, we decided to move on. We would write better songs.

Afterwards Ritchie and I vowed to become more professional. We called a band meeting in the Granary pub to announce that we were going to stamp out people showing up late for rehearsals or recordings. Another new rule was that anyone who took the stage while they were out of their tree would be thrown out of the band. The guitarists had to buy tuners for their guitars and from now on we would rehearse in the mornings. We dumped any song that had a minor chord in it. Furthermore, we made a rule that there would be no more fiddly bits in the middle of sax solos. We insisted that Bozo get a new van, one that had a working accelerator cable as well as windows in the back – we were sick of playing cards in the dark on the way back from gigs. Bozo was also instructed to quit his habit of overtaking while removing his jacket. Finally, we banned all girlfriends from travelling in the van. We were not a 'picnic' band.

Instead of focusing everyone's mind on the band, the new regime simply focused everyone's mind on what they hated about everyone else.

The result was vicious bickering accompanied by threats of physical violence. I told The Individual that he was talking rubbish. 'Shut up or I'll rip your face off,' I shouted. A chair was kicked over. The owner of the pub had to ask us to calm down or leave. In the end, we reached a compromise – we fired Dangerous Abe.

The next morning, Dangerous Abe took the news badly. We dropped him at the side of the road on our way to a gig. He looked sad and fed up. Before we pulled away he called on us to wait. He had something important he needed to say to us. 'You guys are making a big mistake. You'll turn into a show band without me.'

★

Our record company phoned to tell us that 'John Wayne' had been arrested in Newry.

'John Wayne' had entered the Irish charts at number twenty-eight. The following week it shot up to number twenty-seven. 'Wayne' sold nearly a thousand copies.

Then the record company ran out of singles.

To save money, the record company had pressed fresh singles in the UK and attempted to smuggle an extra three hundred of them into the country via Belfast without paying import duty. The police will be looking for IRA men and guns, the record company guy had reasoned, they won't bother with a few singles.

Customs had searched the car, discovered one thousand three hundred copies of 'John Wayne' with a customs form indicating that the record company guy had been given clearance to import a thousand and the lot was promptly impounded, including the car. The record company guy was lucky not to wind up in jail.

Now another record company guy was on his way to Newry to make an attempt to get the car back.

'What about "John Wayne"?' I asked.

'Oh yeah, that too,' he said.

The others were shocked when I told them the news.

'Our first hit is a miss,' Wong said.
'It's like getting to number eleven in the Top Ten,' Ritchie said.
'This fucking band is jinxed,' The Lizard said.
I began to think that The Lizard was right.

★

Extract from Rocky's diary
January 1982

We played brilliantly at The Sportsman's on Sunday night. However, there was one small problem in the form of a decibel meter, installed by the local residents' association to control the noise from those awful loud rock bands. The decibel meter was a special bulb that had been inserted directly above the stage. The bulb was connected to a microphone halfway down the room. Whenever the noise went above ninety-five decibels, the light bulb turned red and the decibel meter at the sound desk cut off all the amplifiers after fifteen seconds. I walked on stage, said 'Hello' into the mic and the red light came on. Ritchie tuned his guitar and the red light came on. No matter how low we kept the volume we still managed to break the sound barrier.

We fought the decibel meter and lost. We were cut off half a dozen times. We handled it all right. We just kept going until the sound returned. Eventually we got fed up and Ritchie and Lizard went into the dressing room and fetched acoustic guitars. We did a dynamite version of 'John Wayne' for the encore. The crowd loved it. At the end of the night, The Egg, our record company guy, climbed on stage and made a speech about how he was never going to allow the band to play The Sportsman's again because of the stupid decibel meter. The red light came on twice during The Egg's speech. He received a sitting ovation.

We played a lunchtime gig on the stage of the Peacock, the little sister to the Abbey Theatre. Our set was a typical Irish farmhouse, complete with kettles and tablecloths and a basket of real eggs. When I was a teenager, Dad had put on a week of special lunchtime gigs featuring Thin Lizzy along with an extract from a play, *The Plebeians Rehearse the Uprising* by Günter Grass. My friends and I had bunked off school to attend each show. At one stage Phil Lynott had upbraided the hippy audience for sneaking off during the play extracts. 'This is fuckin' culture, so stay and watch it and we'll be back on stage in half an hour.'

Now here I was, in the centre of Dad's world. I wondered if he would come to see us. He hadn't thought much of my quitting RTÉ to go full time with a new band. He had figured that I'd got all that stuff out of my system with the Gravediggers. Now he'd see that I was fulfilling myself. Maybe he would understand that I was trying to do my own kind of theatre. (Dad was there, but he didn't say hello and I didn't find out that he had seen our performance for many years.)

It was a really good gig. For some reason, Clint showed up dressed as a New York cop. Mother came to the gig, as did my brother, Niall. Brush Shiels showed up. Brush had taught Phil Lynott to play bass. He had also been bass player with the original Skid Row, featuring Gary Moore. In the late sixties, Skid Row had scored chart success in England and the US. Then Gary Moore had left and the band had experienced mixed fortunes ever since. Brush was funny and wise and insightful. He never used drink or drugs. He didn't have to because he was permanently high on life itself. Brush had once claimed that he was a better guitarist than Jimi Hendrix. He had explained that there were millions of people who were better guitarists than Hendrix, and he just happened to be one of them. After the gig I asked him what he thought. He told us that we were a good blues boogie band with some OK songs. 'At times you're brilliant,' he smiled, 'but even when you're brilliant, you're not as brilliant as you think you are.'

I took Brush's comments as a good review from a legend.

Bozo got a new van, a big brand-new blue Mercedes with air conditioning and power steering and a tape deck, but still no windows in the back. Bozo hated his nickname, so everyone got a great kick out of the new van's registration, which contained the letters 'OZO'. Travelling anywhere at night was grim. We still had to play cards in the dark. Every time the van turned a corner all the money ended up on the floor.

Then Bozo decided that he should receive an extra 'whack' whenever the band made money on a gig. Ritchie and I sat in Bozo's big blue Mercedes van outside my apartment for hours arguing about his 'whack'.

The next day, Bozo said to forget the 'whack', he wanted a regular wage plus expenses – and a 'bonus' whenever we did well. That 'bonus' would be determined by him, but we would not find him unreasonable, he was open to deferred payments, though he would probably have to charge interest because he wasn't a charity. I told him to forget it. He would get paid his agreed fee and that was it, no more. Bozo said that everyone else had agreed to his plan. I was the big problem in the band. He said I was an egotist. 'You deserve to get an iron bar shoved up your sphincter,' he told me.

At a bar in County Cork, the barman showed us to our dressing room, a private lounge. He placed a tape in the video recorder of a large TV and pressed the play button. 'Here's a little something to relax you, lads,' he winked and left us.

The 'little something' turned out to be *Swedish Erotica Volume 3*, a porno movie that featured the most graphic sex acts that any of us had ever witnessed and some that we had never imagined or heard about. It was the first porno film I had ever watched and I was gobsmacked, but not particularly aroused. The naked couplings seemed remote yet oddly natural, as though this was what sex in Sweden was really like – lots of high energy but extremely polite shagging in cold bedsits and dingy hotel rooms. There was a mammoth sex session on a deserted film set between a female 'director' and a leading man as they 'rehearsed' the next day's scene. An hour later, when we received our cue to go on stage, we rose sluggishly, turned off the TV and staggered out to the stage, battling to get the images out of our heads. Wong was the most deeply affected. 'I just need a few moments,' he said. 'I can't walk.'

After Lisdoonvarna and another Macroom, we stayed with Noel Redding again. In the morning Redding invited me to a Sunday afternoon music session in a local pub, Shanleys. He played guitar as I sang a version of Roy C's 'Shotgun Wedding', 'John Wayne' and Donnie Elbert's soul classic 'Little Piece of Leather'. It was one of the warmest and most satisfying gigs I have ever played.

Afterwards we drove back to his house along long, twisting back roads. 'We might do something one day,' he said. 'You should think about it.' I said that I would be interested, but I wanted to see what was going to happen with The Rhythm Kings. I told him I could never leave the band. 'Yes, I know,' he said, 'but you can never tell. I thought that I would never leave Hendrix, but look what happened.'

★

Wong began to forget parts of his drum kit. He left a tom-tom in Navan. He forgot a cymbal in Roundwood. He said it wasn't his fault. We didn't give him time to knock down his kit properly. No wonder he was always forgetting stuff. Ritchie said it was because Wong still hadn't recovered from *Swedish Erotica Volume 3*.

The Individual left his sax in Donegal. Half the band showed up late for a live recording at RTÉ. Ritchie missed

some gigs due to illness. Clint and I had a series of disagreements over musical direction, busy bass-playing and finally
songwriting. We had a bad falling out about who had written
what parts of what songs. Everyone had a go at The Individual.
We were tired and grumpy and broke and Bozo's new van still
kept breaking down on the way to and from gigs.

After a year, the band was falling apart.

At a gig in a country ballroom, our new soundman, Jim Bob,
decided to demonstrate his superior strength by balancing an
immense sound desk over his head on one hand. He managed
the feat for about five seconds before abruptly dropping the
sound desk onto the floor, where it detonated with an almighty
crash. 'I don't know how much more of this I can take,' Ritchie
said. 'This band seems to attract every looper in the country.'

We convened yet another emergency band meeting in the
Granary pub. Ritchie and I had compiled a list of war crimes
– but the rest of the band had also compiled a list.

Within five minutes the band meeting had become an argument that embraced lateness (The Individual, Clint), greedy
van drivers (Bozo), egotistical assholes (me), sloppy management (Ritchie), musical differences (me), crappy stage wear
(Lizard), bad attitude (everyone) and the stupidity of booking
and playing those fucking useless ballroom gigs (Ritchie and I
were jointly indicted).

We argued for hours and got nowhere. Nobody admitted to
any of the war crimes. The Lizard, who had been sitting quietly all night, was criticised for his lack of dress sense and he
snapped. Immediately, he stood up and went into a rant. 'Let's
get this straight. We have a singer who can't sing, a rhythm guitarist with no sense of rhythm, a snobby bass player, a sax guy
who's always out of his skull and a drummer who leaves bits of
his kit all over the country and you think that this band has
problems because of my jacket?'

In the end, we reached the only solution possible. We decided to fire Bozo for driving us in a van that had no windows in back. We gave him a week's notice at the next gig, but Bozo refused to go. He lobbied the others. He called me names. He started a petition to keep him on as driver. He said it would be better if I left because I was the one holding the band back.

'Oh yeah?' I said. 'Who'll do the singing if I leave?'

'Anyone would sing better than you.'

'Why are we wasting all this time fighting with our van driver?' Clint asked.

I had no answer to that.

★

One day I was phoned at home and invited to contest a forth-coming by-election in County Clare against Síle de Valera. The caller was Billy Loughnane, whose late father, Dr Bill, had held the seat for many years.

'You see, Rocky De Valera would come before Síle's name on the ballot sheet,' he explained. 'There's a hell of a lot of peo-ple down here who'd love to see that happen.' He also said that it would be guaranteed good craic.

I said that I would consider giving it a shot. For a few days I fantasised about fighting and winning the election. I would become a TD. I would have power. A chauffeur-driven State limo would take me to gigs. I could introduce new bills. I could legalise fist-fighting in the Dáil.

Then Billy phoned back to say that he had decided to con-test the by-election himself. Would the band come down to play a gig for him? I was disappointed that I wasn't going to become a power broker, but I got over it the instant Billy promised that the band would receive a handsome fee for the gig.

A week later we drove down to Clare in the minibus driven by our new driver, Poindexter. Poindexter didn't drink or smoke, but his idea of a good time was to overtake juggernauts on a bend with his eyes shut. He said it improved his other senses. He believed in keeping one's wits sharpened for life's continual struggle.

The political-rally-cum-rock-concert took place in a glossy hotel in the middle of Ennis. On the way in we passed two men in the reception area who were wearing large Fine Gael rosettes. The men were arguing loudly about me.

'I tell you, he's the young De Valera who is always in trouble up in Dublin,' one said.

'Nonsense,' the other man said. 'He's a chancer who's chancing his arm.'

'Well, I heard he was Síle's brother.'

'No, he's a De Valera all right, but not from this country.'

We met Val, Billy's campaign manager, and asked him if Billy was going to get in. 'No,' he replied. 'But neither will Síle.'

Everyone thought that Billy was a great character. They reckoned he had 'some neck' for going up at all.

The gig started at ten to twelve. We took the stage without having met the man himself, who was out canvassing. Of the six hundred people crammed into the hall, only about six were sober and at least half of those were on stage. The gig became noisier and wilder. People swung from the rafters above us. Others climbed onto the PA stacks to throw themselves into the heaving crowd.

Around halfway through, a wild-eyed, curly-haired figure scrambled onto the stage. The figure came up to me and stuck out his hand. 'Hi, I'm Billy Loughnane.'

I gathered from his disposition and his slight swaying motions that he had come to introduce himself, make a brief speech and maybe join in a song or two. Another clue that Billy wanted to make a speech came when he swiftly grabbed the microphone from my grasp and began yelling into it.

We brought the music down to a soft twelve-bar shuffle.

Billy's arms made wild, windmilling movements as he spoke. 'I want all of you to vote for all of me. I want each and every one of you to go out and find me ten others who'll do the same. Ireland needs the votes of its young people and it needs them now.'

Everything Billy said brought forth enormous cheers. He finished his speech and had a go at singing 'Mean Woman Blues'. Everyone agreed that as a singer he made a great politician. His speeches were more musical.

At the party afterwards upstairs in the Queen's Hotel, Billy made more speeches and was wildly applauded and toasted. The concert was deemed a great success. At one stage Billy and a bunch of his canvassers went into a communal hug, to the disgust of The Lizard. 'I thought we were playing for a real character,' he said. 'But he's just another fucking hippy.'

In the early hours I got into a long conversation with one of Billy's election canvassers, who enquired about the health of my sister. I told him that to the best of my knowledge my sister was fine, whereupon the man rose and shook my hand. 'I hope Billy gets in, but I hope your sister gets in as well.' Which is when it dawned on me that the canvasser had presumed that Síle de Valera was my sister.

As it happened, Billy didn't get elected, but neither did 'my sister'.

★

As a result of my new notoriety, I was offered a three-week stint as a panellist on *The Late Late Show*. It felt odd to be going back to the show as a guest instead of a researcher.

I was teamed with Terri Prone, a smart and funny media guru and writer. Before going on air, Gay said that he was 'expecting great things' from the pair of us.

On the first night I slagged off a new burglar alarm that was reputed to be loud enough to frighten away burglars. 'What if the burglar is deaf?' I asked, and took it from there.

Bono came on to talk about the success of U2. He wore a mullet haircut with a white badger stripe through the centre. He talked about meeting Garret FitzGerald (the leader of Fine Gael) and attempting to discuss politics, but he thought that Garret hadn't taken him seriously. I told Bono that it might have been because of the dead badger he was wearing on his head. He took the slagging with good grace. I had taken him aside in hospitality beforehand and told him that I was going to make smartass remarks about his haircut. He had told me to go ahead, but he still didn't explain why he was wearing a dead badger on his head. The new panel was a big hit.

Something happened to my confidence after that night. Because of the attention and acclaim, I felt exposed in a way that I had never experienced before. I had difficulty coming to terms with being recognised in the corner shop or yelled at from cars. This was my first real taste of fame, and I didn't like it. My privacy was gone. I clammed up after the first week and made very little contribution as a panellist for the remaining shows. The *Late Late* retained us for an extra week, but that was more a tribute to Terri's TV skills than mine.

I found it ironic that I had become extremely famous at the same time as being totally broke. I had become better known as a talk-show panellist than as a rock and roller.

The band was bringing in very little money. I was basically living off Jenny and whatever I could scrounge from writing occasional freelance articles for the newspapers or magazines. I realised that I was no longer an observer. I was now a participant.

The result of my four-week stint on the *Late Late* was that I became the best-known pauper in Ireland.

★

Extract from Rocky's diary
Belfast, Friday, 13 December 1982

*Today we played Queen's. It wasn't Friday the 13th for
nothing.*

*Before the gig some of the students warned us where to go, or
rather, where not to go, for drinks. 'Don't go there – all the
UDA boys drink in that place. Don't go to that bar either – a
lot of rough boys go there. Once they hear that accent, you'll
find out that you're in the wrong place at the wrong time.'*

*It was reassuring to have so many people looking out for us.
Wong said that I should change my name to Abdul Ben Habib.
The gig was magical, but after we had packed away the gear,
we discovered that the clutch cable in the van had died. We cut
cards to see who would travel back in The Individual's car and
who would have to remain in Belfast until the van got fixed.
Clint drew a king. I drew the ten of hearts. Ritchie got the ten
of clubs. Wong drew a five and groaned. Lizard, slowly and
timidly, pulled out a three of diamonds. We climbed into The
Individual's car, waving goodbye to Wong and Lizard and
ignoring their final entreaties to switch places with anyone in
the car for a tenner.*

*We left Belfast and got home in just over two hours. You
always know when you've crossed the border. Even at night,
when you barely notice the customs post, there is a sudden
feeling of uplift, like a convict on his way to the chair who is
granted a reprieve. We have never encountered any personal
antagonism or unpleasantness in the North. All the same,
there is always a sense of violence in the air, like something is
about to go off.*

*At the back of my mind, I nurse a recurring nightmare – a
roadblock in front of us in the middle of nowhere. A hooded
face at the window gently rasping in a soft Northern lilt, 'OK,
which one of you is Rocky DeValera? Step out of the van for a*

moment, please.' Bang! Bang! That's the kind of nightmare you can do nothing about until it's too late, as the Miami Showband discovered when they were stopped at a bogus checkpoint by loyalist paramilitaries [who then opened fire, killing several of the musicians, including the famous singer, Fran O'Toole].

Ritchie said it was a good job we played the gig in Queen's and went down a bomb (ouch).

We released a new single, a ballad, 'Baby, Don't You Worry About a Thing'. People said nice things about the song. RTÉ put 'Baby' on their playlist. My *Late Late* fame ensured that we received maximum coverage in all the country papers. This song would definitely establish the band and bring us that important big hit. It would get us an album deal.

We received good reviews. The record began to sell. This was the one, the breakthrough. There was talk of making an album. I was confident that we had cracked it. Then we did an interview on Radio Nova, a pirate station.

The following day, RTÉ dropped 'Baby' from the playlist. We had committed radio suicide by allowing ourselves to be interviewed by an illegal radio station. There was nothing we could do. 'Baby', which had been bubbling under the Top Twenty, vanished. The ban was overturned a month later but by then it was too late. 'Baby' eventually became an 'airplay hit', a polite way of saying that nobody bought it.

We responded by doing more ballroom gigs and by fighting amongst ourselves. I fought with everyone, even Lizard. I felt insecure. My big dream was melting. I blamed myself, but I blamed everyone else as well.

After a gig in Galway, I went out to Inverin in Connemara to visit my mother. My parents had sold the house in Howth some years before and moved to Connemara with my brother Niall and my little sister Darina, who was known as Doll. I had felt a jagged pain in my stomach when I heard that the house in Howth was gone. I had ambivalent feelings about Howth, but I still saw that white-walled bungalow as my home. Now new people lived in my old house. I wondered if the new people had changed the house much. I wondered if they had repaired the gates and cleared away the white-painted stumps that for years had stood at the bottom of our driveway like underfed sentries.

The new house in Inverin was a former police barracks. It had fine wooden beams and white walls, but it didn't feel like a home to me. Mother and I talked for a while. She wondered when I was thinking of giving up the band and taking a job. I told her that the band was doing fine. 'Yes,' she said, drawing on her cigarette. 'I though you might say that.'

She didn't mention Jenny, who she didn't like. She told me I should get in touch with Dad sometime and I said I would, but I didn't. I didn't know what to say to him. I felt that I needed to make a big success of the band before I could reconnect with my father. He and I hadn't fallen out, we had drifted apart, ending up with nothing much to say to one another.

★

I argued with Clint and drove him mad. Minor problems became huge in my head. Clint decided to quit, but agreed to play on until we finished the tour commitments. The band divided. Wong and The Individual sat at the bar with Clint before a gig. Lizard and Ritchie drank pints with me. Each side moaned about the other. Clint showed up for each gig at the last possible moment, bass guitar slung over his back like a rifle. He wore a curious expression, as though he was really someplace else. I knew that I had hurt him and that I should go up to him and apologise, but I was too obstinate. I told myself that Clint leaving was a good thing. I knew I was lying to myself. Clint's last gig with the band was a sad affair. I shook hands with him afterwards, but it felt like an empty, pathetic gesture, an opportunity missed and a good friend lost.

We recruited a new bassist, Shea Stadium. Shea was a good musician and a nice guy, if a trifle vague about things. But something always felt wrong. For months afterward I kept turning around on stage expecting to find Clint plucking out bass lines, looking cool and aloof in his blind-man's shades with a lit cigarette bobbing in his mouth.

We got a new manager, Meatloaf, and fired him after six months. We played innumerable gigs where the promoter ripped us off, sometimes for as little as fifteen pounds. A favourite trick of the promoter's was to leave while we were on stage, leaving a sum far below our agreed fee with the bouncers. You don't argue about anything with bouncers.

We fired Wong for continuing to leave parts of his kit all over the country, replacing him with our new driver, Luggage, who had once played with The Vipers. The Individual left and came back a couple of times. We threw him out, but he refused to go. The Individual always managed to hang on in there. 'The line-up of this band is about as stable as the Irish economy,' Ritchie said. The Individual was likeable and talented. On a good night, he was one of the best harmonica players in the world and he could be a more than adequate saxophonist. The trick was to get him on stage or into the studio on a good night. I could never understand how he could practise all day and then get completely banjaxed before going on stage. One night at the Stables in Greystones he was so out of it that during the first few numbers he sang backing vocals into the clip of a microphone stand, failing to notice that he had knocked the microphone onto the floor. Halfway through the gig, he collapsed into his own saxophone case.

★

Somehow we managed to get an album deal from Scoff. Everything now hinged on the success of our album. The record company put up six grand for the recording. We hired a producer who told us that we were a great band with great songs.

On the third day of recording, we fell out with the producer. Then we argued with the record company about falling out with the producer. We fired The Individual for turning up drunk to a recording session, but then realised that we needed him to finish the album so we hired him back. The next morning, he turned up drunk and we fired him again. One morning our engineer had to go to a funeral. His replacement accidentally wiped out half of one of our songs. Tempers became frayed. There were arguments.

One morning Lizard and Ritchie swore that they had heard a mysterious guitar playing on certain songs during a playback. Someone had been sneaking into the studio to overdub guitar parts on our songs for our album. The producer denied all knowledge. The record company said they didn't know what we were talking about. I watched through the control studio glass as Ritchie and Lizard confronted the producer about the 'mystery guitar'. The producer said that there had been no 'mystery guitar', but now that they mentioned it, wouldn't it be a really good idea to hire a session guitarist to overdub some of the guitar tracks? Particularly those tracks that were 'a bit lacking', which in effect meant most of them. Relations between the guitar section and the record producer broke down irretrievably.

The Individual turned up drunk again. We argued with him, threatened to fire him and even offered to put him up in the studio overnight under guard so that he would be sober the next morning, but nothing worked. The Individual's girlfriend had gone back to Paris and he missed her.

By a miracle, we finished recording the album.

★

Extract from Rocky's diary
London, 8–13 November 1982

Right now I'm on my way home from the Big Smoke with the multi-reels of the new album. Ritchie is asleep opposite me and this infernal train journey just drags on. Years ago, I swore that I would never again travel by boat and train to London and back. But this time there were economic reasons (we spent all the money on the album) that necessitated Ritchie and I taking the cheap route. I find myself at twenty-seven years of age, repeating the pattern of my college years as I struggle to get comfortable on these hideous train seats. The voyage over was boring, except for Ritchie turning white and vanishing to the jax for an hour or so. When he returned he announced that he hadn't 'delivered the goods' but that he had taken a pill and should be fine now…

London hadn't changed much. Still the same brassy, suspicious city, full of scrumptiously dressed women and arrogant taxi drivers. Ritchie insisted on wearing that dreadful white Inspector Clouseau mac everywhere we went. He wouldn't take it off, even when I refused to walk down the street with him. His attitude was that there was no way he was going to catch a cold in London. But he did.

The heaters in our hotel room were turned up full and couldn't be switched off, a fact that made Ritchie even more unwell and ensured that he only got a couple of hours sleep a night.

The studio was under an archway in Little Russell Street, off Oxford Street. It was small, homely and comfortable. Ritchie said we should move into the control room and sleep there instead. Kenny Jones was the engineer – super-cool, super-efficient, quiet and very obviously an almost recovered hippy.

Every mix took almost three hours to complete. We were bored silly. By the third day of mixing, we had taken to going for long walks or to the movies. We saw The Loveless *with Willem Dafoe and Robert Gordon. There wasn't a speck on any of the shiny leather jackets throughout the whole film. Gordon was good, though, and he sang great versions of Jack Scott songs. That night we hustled tickets for Squeeze's farewell concert. It was magnificent. Marvellous songs, impeccable harmony singing, brilliant musicianship and sheer professionalism (though a complete absence of charisma). Best lightshow I have ever seen. They taught us a lot of lessons. Dave Edmunds came on for the encore and did some rock and roll. Ritchie went bananas, jumping up and down yelling, 'Fucking great, fucking great.' He may profess to be a cynic, but deep down he's still a little kid whose biggest kick is getting to see his heroes live in the flesh on stage.*

The next morning, Rebop, who played congas with Traffic, strolled into the studio while we were mixing our version of '54–46, That's My Number'. 'Say man,' he said to me. 'What's the name of your group?'

'The Rhythm Kings,' I told him.

'Yes, sir, man, you are The Rhythm Kings,' Rebop said, and wandered out.

We went to see The Belle Stars. They were awful. Out of tune, the singer couldn't sing, their sound was desperate and if it hadn't been for the two-piece brass section (two saxes) they would have been a total dead loss. I was glad to see, though, that an English band with two Top Twenty chart hits could still suffer from appalling sound problems.

We completed the mix on Thursday evening. We spent Friday morning listening to it. Everyone was pleased. The album is slightly laid-back and that is a bit of a shock. I hope it comes as a pleasant surprise to those who have no time for the band.

Ritchie and I left London on Friday evening (after going to see Flesh Gordon, *a comic porn version of the obvious).We felt good about things, despite the fact that we were laden down with master tapes and multi-reels. The journey home was the usual slog that I remembered so well from student days.*

In the beginning we all said we loved the album, except Luggage, who said that he wasn't sure what he was hearing. 'Is that us? It doesn't sound like us.'

The album received good reviews and reached number four in the Top Ten albums in Dublin.

After two weeks, the album sank rapidly off the charts. A week later we began to go off our masterpiece, even despised it. At the end of a month, nearly everyone said they had hated it from the moment they'd heard it but had kept their mouths shut because they didn't want to hurt anyone's feelings. Most of the songs now sounded like bath water going down a drain. There seemed to be no treble register. Everything came across as muddy and dull. My vocals sounded thin and exposed. I had a limited vocal range, but the album made me sound as though I had no vocal range. The guitars sounded like bed-springs.

The Atrix made a better album. Some Kind of Wonderful released a better single. Tokyo Olympics moved to London. U2 began to break big in America. The Bogey Boys drew huge audiences whenever they played. The Blades always got rave reviews in *Hot Press*.

I went to see The Lookalikes in the Baggot. The audience was ninety-nine per cent women, beautiful women who stared at the stage while The Lookalikes played. The Lookalikes were very obviously the best-looking band around. They looked sharp and they had good songs as well. The mullet-headed bastards.

I left the Baggot feeling profoundly depressed.

Despite the terrible economic situation and the mass unemployment, the nightclubs in Dublin were always full. On a Monday night there was usually a good crowd in any of them – Brats, The Pink Elephant or Risks. We now inhabited a world where nobody had a real name. Our booking agent was Louis Walsh, known as 'Big Louis' because he was impossibly boyish and smiley. Big Louis enjoyed hearing about our antics on the road. Sometimes he waived his ten per cent booking fee in return for us dropping in to see him to relate tales of our wild shenanigans, the fist-fights, arguments and name-calling, van breakdown disasters and the rest of the mayhem that accompanied everything we did. He came to see us at The Sportsman's. He said we were a good band but we needed to do more Chuck Berrys.

Our new manager was also the boss of our record company, Scoff. We called him 'The Egg' because of his baldness. He made us promise to give him at least six months before we fired him. We were offered a two-day tour of Fiji. We declined because we would have to pay our own air fares. We also turned down a gig in East Berlin. We had enough trouble trying to get to Strokestown or Moate. Nobody in their right mind would send this band to East Berlin, let alone Fiji. There were no offers of a gig in London. We carried on touring the country like mindless hedonists.

We hung around with friends like Goalpost, Mixer and the Hyena along with the Hyena's brother, the Young Hyena. The girls we dated had nicknames as well – The Spirit Woman (because she kept seeing the ghost of Richard Brinsley Sheridan everywhere), The Waif (because she was), Dallas Alice (because it rhymed), Piranha (she preferred biting to kissing), Ponytails from Ballaghaderreen (most elaborate ponytails anyone had ever seen), Detroit Sue (from Detroit), Tiger Woman (wore tiger-skin miniskirts) and Vampirella (she liked to bite your neck till she tasted blood).

Drugs were around and nearly always free for any musician who wanted them. Most of us preferred to drink. Beer at the gig usually followed by cheap wine in a nightclub afterwards or if we could afford it, champagne. We don't have a drink problem we told everyone – we drink, we get drunk, there's no problem.

One night I ran into Colm Tóibín in Wylde's. As features editor of *In Dublin*, he had commissioned some articles from me about the adventures of The Rhythm Kings that had been well received. Now he had just taken over at *Magill*. He promised to throw some work my way. I knew that he wrote short stories. I asked him if he had written any fiction lately. 'No,' he said. 'Have you?'

'No,' I replied, and I knew that I wasn't likely to the way things were going. Tóibín was working and living in the real world. I was an astronaut from a Ray Bradbury story, free-falling through space after a spaceship wreck.

We played a gig as support to Bo Diddley at UCD Fresher's Ball. Bo laughed at all our nicknames. He thought The Lizard was a really good guitarist. We shared a plate of fried chicken. 'That's exactly where it's at,' Bo Diddley said. 'Where I come from, we call this gospel bird.'

'Where I come from,' Lizard said, 'we eat anything.'

Gradually, the real world of day jobs and normal life slid away to be replaced by almost permanent night-time. I rarely saw mornings, and if I did it was usually through the windows of a van on our way back to Dublin. The nights went on forever. In one nightclub gangsters hung out and mingled with clubbers and I once watched a gangster from a prominent Dublin crime family fall asleep on the counter at the tiny bar. His jacket opened and a pistol fell out and slid out onto the small dance floor. A Midge Ure lookalike casually picked up the pistol and put it back in the sleeping gangster's pocket, and then he went back to the dance floor to continue bopping to

'Pull Up to the Bumper' by Grace Jones. It seemed perfectly normal to me at the time.

I drank too much and I knew I was drinking too much. I stopped several times, but there was always an excuse to get hammered at the next gig or the crucial band meeting or the next recording session or after we had just thrown someone out of the group. Sometimes, after a lot of pints, I snorted lines of coke. The only effect it had on me was to make me think I was sober. That meant I could drink more. I didn't like drugs. Once I snorted some weird stuff on the way to a gig and collapsed in the van. The Individual revived me and walked me around. The band referred to the incident as 'The Day Rocky Died'. After that, I mostly stuck to drink – at least you didn't have to put Guinness up your nose to feel the effect. Jenny worried about me. She told me I was becoming very self-destructive. I quit drinking and we made plans to go to Paris – to quit Dublin and walk away from the band and leave everything. That lasted until the next gig.

In Belfast we played on the same bill as Gary Glitter. I fell off the high stage and grabbed hold of Gary Glitter's special stage curtain, splitting it in two all the way to the bottom, like Harpo Marx in *A Night at the Opera*. It took me ages to climb back on stage to realise that the band hadn't noticed I had fallen, or even that I'd left the stage. Later, Gary Glitter had us moved from our dressing room. He wanted all other artists cleared from his backstage area so that he could make his big entrance. Gary's big entrance didn't seem so big when they hoisted his special curtain only to discover that it was torn in half.

★

I started seeing Della, a beautiful girl from Bray who was almost as tall as me. The relationship ended one night after a gig when Della gave me a lift and crashed her brand-new Datsun Cherry into the back of a car that was parked on the corner of a wet road. I stood in the road with an umbrella and a flashlight while the band and the road crew and all of the people who had been at the gig drove past with their faces pressed to the window, wondering why Rocky De Valera was standing in the middle of the road in the lashing rain behaving like a traffic light.

To liven up our stage show I recruited Lesley, a petite, extremely pretty girl with an elfin face and a big voice who had been lead singer with a band that supported us in the Baggot Inn. Lesley recorded a demo of new songs with the band. Then she came on the road with us, singing back-up and sharing lead vocals on half a dozen songs, including the encores. We played some sensational live gigs with Lesley. Whenever I introduced Lesley as 'our little sister, Síle', the crowd went mad.

Ritchie fell in love with Lesley. His expressions as he snatched looks at her on stage or in the van or at rehearsals or when we were in the dressing room were truly tragic to behold. Then Luggage started going out with Lesley, and Ritchie stopped talking to Luggage. I was mad at Luggage too, because I had been waiting for my chance to make a move on Lesley. I had waited too long, and now I was pissed off. I quit talking to Luggage, too but Luggage didn't notice because he was too busy hanging out with his new girlfriend.

One night Lizard took me aside after a gig to inform me that the band was falling to bits because most of the band members were either in love with Lesley, obsessed with Lesley or going out with Lesley. The result was that nobody was talking to any-one and he thought the band was going to self-destruct if someone didn't do something fast. I didn't tell Lizard that I also fancied Lesley. Instead I thanked him for the information and told him I'd work something out.

That night I agonised about what to do. Lesley had done nothing wrong; in fact, she had been a major attribute to the band. With her, we had played some of the best gigs of our career. Now I was going to have to fire her because of the unbridled lust and passions and jealousy that her presence stirred within the band. We were turning into Fleetwood Mac, only without the hit songs.

The next day, I told Lesley the truth. I apologised and told her that we had to let her go because of the way her presence was affecting the band. She took the news really well. Perhaps it was a relief to her. She gave me a kiss on the cheek and a big hug and told me that singing with the band had been a wonderful experience. She had never seen it as a long-term thing anyhow.

Afterwards I felt as though I was the one who had just been let go.

★

Once he had gotten over his infatuation with Lesley, Ritchie became a woman magnet. He metamorphosed from a shy nice and slightly awkward guy into the band's resident Casanova. Beautiful girls went out of their way to get him. Lizard said that Ritchie was 'dripping with women'.

I got back together with Jenny again, then we broke up, then we got back together again. Our 'open' relationship didn't work, but somehow we remained friends even though I didn't know what I was doing. I felt more comfortable with one-night stands or short flings than with an intimate, long-term relationship.

I didn't know what I wanted from my relationship, from the band or from life. I didn't write songs anymore. I didn't listen to music either. I couldn't read, I kept hearing loud, distorted guitars playing in my head.

I felt as though I was water-skiing barefoot. However, I seemed to be keeping my balance for an awfully long time. I thought I was indestructible. Even though I kept catching colds and flus and sore throats that lasted for weeks, I believed that I would live forever. I convinced myself that the band would make it and everything would work out well in the end. In the meantime, we played meaningless gigs, broke down, drank too much, fought amongst ourselves and had mad, quite brilliant fun while enjoying many fantastic nights on stage where sometimes the music connected and made exhilarating, beautiful sense, once again exciting and inspiring me, reminding me why I had chosen to get into this crazy business.

The band became my life. The band was my food and drink and oxygen. The band was my spiritual base. I ate my breakfast in the Stella Maris guesthouse. I dined in the Del Rio Café. I attended religious services in The Bananas Club in Dundalk, Sir Henry's in Cork, Alice Kyteler's pub in Kilkenny and Tingles Ballroom, Ballaghderreen. Mecca was the Baggot Inn. When we crossed the border into Northern Ireland, the young squaddies who checked our van were fans of Dr Feelgood and Spandau Ballet, not soldiers who carried real rifles. The paramilitary club owner who paid us in sterling and then winked while he revealed the semi-automatic in his waistband, telling us we were always safe while we were on his premises, was just another character from Dublin's nightlife. The convicted murderer I met at the bar before a gig at the Baggot Inn who had sworn never to carry a knife again after seeing The Specials at The Olympia struck me as a nice guy.

We stayed with Redding again. He was in bad form because his struggle to reclaim his royalties from all the Hendrix recordings had run into more snags. 'It's all lawyers, man,' he said. 'It's not about music at all.' I had never seen him so down. We made plans to meet up in Dublin, but somehow we never did.

In Bandon we played a three-night residency. We noticed a large glass chandelier hanging in the foyer. Going up the stairs it was possible to reach over and remove the chandelier's glass ornaments. The ornaments had tiny hooks and made wonderful earrings. We hung the glass pieces from our ears and marched about like eastern princes. When people complimented us on our wonderful earrings, we told them where they could get some. That night nearly everyone in our audience sported a glass earring. By the second night the hotel chandelier was reduced to a thin framework of hanging bulbs. The hotel staff must have noticed, but they didn't let on. People saw the world differently in Bandon.

The band continued to change line-ups, but I didn't care. We gave up rehearsing and writing new songs. I tried to learn to play the guitar, but I couldn't grasp it. It was as though I was back in Coláiste Mhuire struggling with algebra.

At a sound check, The Individual wasted hours getting odd sounds from his harmonica or sax. 'I want you to make my harmonica sound like a concrete block landing on someone's head,' he instructed our soundman.

We gave up doing sound checks. Soon after that, The Individual quit. Then he rejoined. After that he quit again, this time for good.

We entered a military phase where everyone in the band was reconfigured in army terms. We became wing commanders, corporals and rear admirals. People we didn't like were addressed as 'Private Parts'. Drinking was 'taking heavy fire'. Gigging was 'instructing the cadets'. Chasing women was known as 'engaging in military manoeuvres'. Failing to score was a 'tactical withdrawal'. Going home alone to bed meant engaging in 'shelling your own troops'.

I missed Clint. I missed his humour and his daft aristocratic dignity. I missed the crazy, meandering but always entertaining arguments and I missed his busy bass playing. Once he went, the soul of the band left with him. I felt guilty for fighting with him and making him quit, but I was too stubborn to ask him to rejoin. I felt as though I had become a rock-and-roll zombie. I started getting drunk before going on stage, something I had always sworn that I would never do.

Somewhere on the road, in some crappy room in some desperate hotel after another pointless drinking session, I got into a stupid argument with Ritchie that ended when I flicked a lit cigarette butt off his nose. Sparks flew. We all sat for a moment as the sparks settled and died on the filthy carpet. Then Ritchie slowly rose and stretched. 'Well, I'm off to bed,' he said and left the room.

I turned to the others. 'It had to be done,' I explained.

Then I conked out.

In the morning, I awoke with the horrors. Immediately, I went and apologised to Ritchie. I had been out of order and stupid. He was very gracious about it.

I was twenty-seven. I had been touring and playing for nearly three years with a rock-and-roll band. I had no fixed income and no pension and no prospects. I felt as though I had had both feet planted firmly in the clouds for a long time. I hadn't made the great record I had wanted to make. All I had really succeeded in achieving was a prolonging of my adolescence. After the incident with the cigarette, I knew it was all over.

A couple of mornings after the cigarette butt throwing, Ritchie and Lizard called around to meet me in my flat in Mountjoy Square. We decided that the band had gone as far as it could and that we should break up. We sat at a table by the window and opened a bottle of brandy that someone had given me as a present. We looked down into the traffic while we chatted about the band and what plans we had for the future and why the whole often miserable and occasionally exhilarating adventure had been worthwhile. I saw Dad's Austin Cambridge pull in at the corner of Mountjoy Square and

Lower Gardiner Street, waiting for a break in the traffic. If he had looked up to the first-floor window of my apartment he would have seen his wayward oldest son drinking brandy with his two closest band mates as though he hadn't a care in the world. But Dad didn't look up. He drove past on his way to the Abbey. I realised that I hadn't seen or spoken to Dad for over three years, as long as The Rhythm Kings had been going.

At noon the bottle was empty but the three of us were still sober. We shook hands and wished each other well.

Our farewell tour lasted six months. To get into the spirit of the thing we decided to sack Shea Stadium, but Shea beat us to it by quitting. Then Shea's replacement quit after a few gigs. Phil from Revolver joined on bass. Now the guy I had once admired as being the epitome of rock-and-roll cool had joined The Rhythm Kings for our farewell tour.

It was the only truly successful period in the band's history. We drew big crowds. The gigs were exciting, the money was good and our van only broke down a couple of times. Ritchie and I speculated on what might happen should we just keep playing a farewell tour. Perhaps we should release farewell singles and a brilliant farewell album. We would have farewell hits, make farewell fortunes.

For our final farewell gig at the Baggot Inn, we hired a limo – it cost thirty pounds but we reckoned it was worth it to exit in style.

★

Extract from Rocky's diary
Saturday, 13 September 1983

We finished up in the Baggot Inn on Friday. The night before we had played Ballybunion, but only after I insisted that we take eighty pounds a man for doing it. I got my way.

Naturally, everyone stayed up all night drinking after the gig. It was a session born of desperation. Nobody really wanted to be there. Phil got on everyone's nerves, continually throwing water and drink about and trying to 'fix' the door handles of all the rooms with shaving cream. Not long to go now, I kept telling myself.

We hit Dublin at around four thirty and stopped off at my place for a shave and wash-up. After a while I got rid of them all and was able to relax.

The others took our hired limo to the Shelbourne, where they drank champagne and were mistaken for first U2 and then Steel Pulse. They signed autographs.

Later we all met in Larry Tobin's, where we drank Charles Heidsieck and posed for photographs for the Evening Press. *Loads of pals turned up and waved us goodbye when the limo (a black Mercedes) came to collect us for the Baggot gig. At the Baggot, more friends applauded our arrival.*

Upstairs in the dressing room, Clint was waiting for us to wish us luck. Nice!

The Baggot was packed and sweaty. The atmosphere was wild and partisan. The gig was a good one. I don't remember much about it now – it all happened too fast, even though we played for two hours and 'swung it' for all we were worth. Tom Matthews the cartoonist passed a note up to me on stage. 'You guys should go professional.'

At the end we ran for it through the crowd. I met Mother at the door on her way in to the gig. She wanted me to go back up on stage and do more. I explained that I couldn't because the gig was over and tears appeared in her eyes. 'Can't you go back and play a song for your own mother? Not even one song?' she asked.

I made some excuse and ran for the dressing room. Upstairs everyone shook hands and embraced. We got one hundred pounds each from the night, the most money we had ever received for a single gig. Then we went downstairs and got into the black limo. Passers-by were saying to each other, 'Who is it? Who are they?'

We barrelled down to The Pink Elephant. I could see that Phil wanted the night to go on forever. Lizard was astonished but enjoying it. Ritchie and Luggage were pissed as newts and determined to get worse. To me, it was all a pleasant dream. Tomorrow, I will wake up to reality, perhaps for the first time in my life.

The Pink brought out a huge cake for us with 'Rhythm Kings' written in chocolate across the top. We drank champagne and ate cake. In half an hour we spent all the money we had laid aside for the night – one hundred and twenty. We started throwing our own money into the fray. 'How much is the champagne?' Lizard asked. He was told that the champagne cost twenty-seven pounds a bottle. 'Is that all?' he cried. 'Give us two.'

We were surrounded by admirers on all sides. We were the absolute focus of attention for everyone in the club. Ritchie scored with a pretty blonde.

Afterwards those of us who could still walk went to Brats and drank there until the bitter end. It was the right way for us to finish. It almost had style.

15

Bald Head

Nobody told me I had cancer. I had to figure it out for myself.

In July 1986 it was just a swelling in my left testicle. No big deal. Most of the time I wasn't even aware of it. There was no pain, just a vague discomfort. I decided it was the result of a kick or a bump and ignored it.

By early August the swelling had increased to the size of a golf ball and turned a bluish-red. Now it was as hard as a stone and a constant irritation. There was still no pain, but sitting down was awkward and crossing my legs a bit of an ordeal.

For a while it seemed as though the extra weight in my pants was causing me to veer to one side when I walked – it was a lot easier to turn to the left than the right. Sometimes I felt like the drunk in an old Charlie Chaplin comedy. It was an embarrassing situation, so I didn't tell anyone.

I kept playing Machoman and reckoned it would go away of its own accord. It never occurred to me that it could be serious. It was just a swelling.

But Kate was worried. She persuaded me to see our local GP, which I finally did, thinking it was a waste of time and mortified that I had to submit to a humiliating examination. The GP diagnosed it as epididymitis and prescribed antibiotics.

A week later the swelling was down, but the discomfort remained.

Throughout the week of the Second Dublin Film Festival – which I attended as part of my job as a film critic, viewing twenty-nine movies – I was forever shifting in my seat, fidgety and uncomfortable no matter how I arranged myself. It was like trying to deal with a rock in your underpants. People sitting behind me must have thought that I really hated the films.

Around that time I met my friend Ritchie in Bewleys. We drank coffee while I told him of my condition in a schoolboy's whisper so that the man sitting across the table couldn't hear. Ritchie thought it was funny. As I explained, I thought it was funny as well. A swollen ball? Epididymitis? It sounded so ridiculous. How could anything bad come from a name as silly as epididymitis? We laughed and dismissed it. The man opposite got so pissed off with our juvenile giggling that he dropped his half-eaten bun into his coffee and left.

But the next morning the testicle had expanded again, and its pinky colour had changed to a dark blood-red. I could barely get out of bed. Getting dressed was no fun at all.

I saw another doctor. This time I was advised to have the problem examined by a specialist, but that week the discomfort eased and so I didn't bother. Machoman would solve his own problems – and besides it looked like the problem was going away.

The following Sunday things suddenly got serious. Kate and I were walking up to the swimming pool of the Killiney Castle Hotel. I had the Sunday papers under my arm and I was doing all right until I got to the corner at the foot of Killiney Hill, where I had to stop. The rock had changed. Now it felt as heavy and cumbersome as a basketball. Every time my leg brushed against it there was pain. 'I can't walk anymore,' I told Kate.

I stood like a flagpole until Kate led me to the bus and brought me home.

That night Kate called our GP, but he was away. His stand-in came over and examined me. He recommended that I go into St Vincent's straightaway to see the specialist.

Kate and I took a taxi to St Vincent's Hospital. On the way we held hands in the back seat. We were both scared and we scarcely said a word. Stupid to feel like this, I thought. It's just a pain in the balls.

★

It had only been a year since the brain haemorrhage, from which I was very lucky to have survived.

Going to hospital again so soon brought back some bad memories, particularly for Kate, who'd spent that weekend waiting around on her own in casualty not knowing if I was going to make it.

I had made it, but it had taken many months for my brain to heal as well as for the shock to wear off. It had been a hard time, though much worse for Kate than for me.

I'd been fortunate. I could have died or been left paralysed down one side of my body or had my memory erased. Instead I made a complete recovery, except for losing my sense of smell, which hadn't returned and probably never will. It was a small price to pay, I reckoned.

Now I was on my way to hospital again. At least this time I was conscious.

Just before we reached St Vincent's, 'Maria' from *West Side Story* came on the car radio. Something bad was coming, I knew. The same song had been playing on the stereo in John and Sally's house the night I'd fallen over. 'Maria' wasn't the kind of song you hear every day. Now it was becoming the theme to our personal disaster movie.

In Vincent's, the night doctor examined me. At one stage he put on a plastic glove and inserted a finger into my rectum. My gasp woke up people who had been dozing on chairs in the waiting room.

After prodding and poking me around the neck and chest, he made an appointment for me to see the specialist the following morning.

Going home in another taxi, I was too stunned to talk much. Kate tried to cheer me up, but there's not much you can say when you're not sure what's going on. I asked the taxi driver to switch off the car radio, just in case some DJ was on a *West Side Story* binge.

The next morning I got to the private clinic early. The specialist was a gruff, sturdy man with the rumbled face of a bloodhound who had seen it all. His face showed only one expression – extreme dissatisfaction. He worked me over thoroughly. Then he arranged for me to go into hospital that night. 'We're going to open you up and have a look,' he said. 'There's a ninety per cent chance that there's nothing there.'

He wasn't the sort of guy you questioned or argued with.

As I was dressing, he phoned the private hospital to reserve a time for surgery. I remember his turning away from me as he spoke softly to the person on the other end of the line. 'It's probably epididymitis, but there's a possibility of a tumour.'

I heard, but it didn't register. When Kate asked me how it went I told her I had to go in for a straightforward examination. No big deal. I even felt relieved. If there had been something seriously wrong, Dr Bloodhound would have told me.

That was Monday. On Tuesday morning I was on the fourth floor of St Vincent's Private Hospital, waiting to be wheeled down to the theatre. They had given me strong drugs to knock me out and I was having one hell of a good time, joking with the nurses.

As the medication took hold, I was left in the care of the older ward sister, who sat across the bed and kept a steady eye on me. We discussed the great success of U2, my work as a journalist and good movies I had seen at the Dublin Film Festival. The last thing I recall is her wide, friendly, dark eyes through her big, round glasses as she slyly studied my face for any sign that the drugs were hitting me the wrong way.

Afterwards I woke up in a white bed. There was no fuzz in my head at all. Everything was clear and still. Sunlight splayed out from the large windows and bathed the whole room. I lifted the top sheet and looked down.

There was a large gauze bandage on my groin. I put my hand down and felt my right testicle, but the left side was numb and my fingers couldn't penetrate the bandage. God, I thought, don't let them have whipped off one of my balls – it must be under the bandage with a big plaster on it. For a second I had a mental image of my left ball in a sling.

I picked up the phone by the bed and dialled home. Kate answered. There were sniffles in her voice. I didn't beat around the bush. 'I lost one, didn't I?'

'Yes love, you did.'

Then she told me they'd found a tumour, a bad one, which had had to come out. I thought about it for a moment. My mind made slow connections. I recalled Dr Bloodhound's phone conversation the day before. 'A tumour? That's cancer, isn't it?'

Kate said that it was cancer. I was to rest and take it easy and she would be in to see me very soon. After that the whole day just seemed to slide away. I don't remember much except holding Kate's hand when she came in and making jokes to try and take the worried look off her lovely, open face. I don't think it worked.

Days later, Kate told me that our GP had let her know that there was a possibility that I had a tumour, but he said it was highly unlikely. It was sure to be just an infection. Besides, it was a billion to one chance that a man my age – just turned thirty-one – could have a brain haemorrhage and cancer within a year. He said he'd call her as soon as he heard from the hospital. So Kate waited at home while they opened me up.

But the second she saw our doctor's car pull up outside the apartment, she knew. When he came inside and told her, she cried. Her mother had died of cancer in 1980. Now her husband could go the same way. First a brain haemorrhage, now cancer. Her Irishman was totally falling to pieces. Kate called my sister, who came over immediately with a bottle of brandy.

Kate and I had met in Dublin in 1984 and had fallen in love almost immediately. Three months after our first date we had married in Kate's summer home, Cape Cod. We had felt young and blessed and invincible. Then less than a year later, I'd started coming apart.

Kate was still crying when I phoned from my hospital bed. She tried to put a brave face on it, but she knew I could feel her distress. As soon as Kate put down the receiver, my sister said, 'That was the greatest performance of your life.'

I'm not sure what I felt after that. It stunned me that I had guessed what was wrong. I had always presumed that a white-coated doctor came to your bedside and gave it to you straight. Either that or a nurse told you. I didn't know that it was medical policy to tell the loved one and let the loved one inform the patient.

Now I was confused. Had the cancer gone completely or was there still some of it left inside me? I didn't understand how it had happened. I figured that I was being punished for something. It made so little sense that I gave up thinking about it and concentrated on what I could see and hear and do and say – the real world, as I saw it then. I had never heard of testicular cancer. The name had a nasty ring to it, so I pushed it out of my mind. I had cancer. That was enough to be worrying about.

When Kate visited the next morning, I joked that there was someone out there with a voodoo doll, sticking pins into my most important parts, doing it systematically. First the brain, then the left ball. Next would come the right ball, followed by the penis…

I tried to think of who might be sticking the pins in the voodoo doll. A former girlfriend? Someone I had let down? One of my enemies? Whoever it was had properly banjaxed Machoman now.

'I'm going to have a badge made,' I said to Kate. 'Back to Mono.'

She gave a tiny laugh.

I didn't think it was funny either.

★

I was never really Machoman, but no man likes to feel that there's anything wrong with his genitalia. Confronting cancer is bad enough, but the possibility of having your manhood taken away is too scary even for nightmares. I didn't know how to face up to either prospect, so I made jokes, deflecting my fears with humour.

For nearly four days after the operation, I couldn't piss. I was in a private room with my own bathroom and toilet. I spent hours standing over the toilet bowl trying to urinate. Nurse Mary had given me a little plastic cup to fill, but I couldn't coax a drop out of my poor, wounded self. From time to time Nurse Mary would call in on me to see how I was getting on, but all I could give her was a silly grin.

So I passed some of the time examining myself in the bathroom. With the puffy white groin bandage and the quaint little elastic jockstrap that held my remaining testicle, I looked like a gladiator who had had a really bad day in the arena. I could feel stitches through the gauze.

The waste fluid was building up in me, but nothing would move it. I tried everything I could think of – running tap water, gentle massage, alternating dips into cups of hot and cold water, even reasoning with my penis in what I hoped were smooth, encouraging tones. Nothing happened, except for a feeling that I was about to burst.

On the morning of the fourth day, I tried all the ploys at once – one immediately after the other. It worked. My urine stream was a beautiful golden brown in the orange bathroom light. It went on for a long time too, which was a great relief, so much so that I forgot about filling the little plastic container.

After that, there was no problem. I could give urine samples almost at will. The only trouble now was that I needed to urinate at least a dozen times a day. In the mornings my bladder felt like a water balloon, sloshing from one side of me to the other. But it was somehow reassuring. It meant that everything was working again.

I was in hospital for two weeks. There were examinations, tests, blood samples, scans and x-rays. It looked pretty good, the doctors said. There was no trace of cancer in my blood or anywhere else in my body.

Dr Bloodhound came to see me. He gave me his usual no-frills examination. He asked me how I was feeling. 'Fine,' I said.

He nodded and pointed to my groin. 'It was very bad. It had to go, had to go.'

I learned later from one of the nurses that Dr Bloodhound in a gruff mood was a good sign. It meant that he was pleased with a patient's progress. If he was nice and smiled a lot, it might mean that you were in big trouble. I liked Dr Bloodhound. I appreciated his no-pussyfooting-around approach.

As the shock of the operation wore off, I began to accept the situation. I had lost one. I still had one. Everyone assured me that there would be no problem. All I had to do was get my strength back and I could resume my life. Kate was optimistic, but she knew that there was a chance that the cancer could reappear.

I kept the news of my operation and stay in hospital as quiet as possible. I didn't want my family to hear of my condition. I told only my editors at work and my friend, Ritchie. Kate and my sister were my only visitors.

But it's hard to keep secrets in Dublin, especially if you've had a high profile for several years.

There were rumours. I'd had a recurrence of the brain haemorrhage. I was a heroin addict. One guy told everyone he met – including my brother Niall – that he'd heard that I had AIDS. Someone else speculated that it was a combination of all three things.

Finally, I was forced to make phone calls from my hospital bed to ask some people I knew to please shut up. Most did, but one man seemed to take great delight in walking up to my friends and acquaintances in pubs, informing them of my illness and then gleefully speculating as to what might be wrong with me. It was just pub talk, but it hurt me at the time.

Somehow we managed to keep the news away from my parents. I would tell them after it was over, I figured, as soon as I was better and back at work.

The two weeks went slowly. Now and again I would find myself thinking about having cancer. Then I would just grow numb and immediately switch to thinking about something else. It was too mysterious and frightening a topic to deal with.

Besides, I thought it was all over. All I had to do now was recover.

During the days there were long visits from Kate. She would tell me what was happening outside, how her work was going, what the doctors were saying. We held hands and I made her laugh. Sometimes she stayed so long that I had to throw her out myself in order to get any sleep.

When it came time for Kate to go, I escorted her to the fourth-floor lifts, where I kissed her goodnight. Then I dashed back to my room to wave to her from the windows. It felt a little like old-style courting, except in reverse. She made me feel very special and much loved. I suppose I made her feel like she was married to a disaster area.

At night I watched pop music on Sky TV. I talked with the nurses, who were always great fun. I read until I got tired. Then I would take a sleeping pill and slowly black out. I don't recall having any dreams at all.

I was discharged in early November. Kate had built new bookshelves in the front room of the apartment and re-arranged the stereo and tape collection. There were flowers in a vase on the kitchen table. It was like walking into a Japanese garden. It made me feel like a prince.

It never occurred to me that the cancer would come back. The doctors had assured me that the problem had been caught and dealt with in time. The cancer had gone, along with my left ball.

I could live with that.

★

I went back to work. Things went well and I felt good, but I could sense that Kate was tentative, worried – the doctors had told her a lot more than they had told me. Deep down, I had a feeling that there was more trouble coming. Every blood test was like an omen.

At Christmas I bought Kate a beautiful black-leather satchel bag, along with as many nice things as I could afford. I wanted to shower presents on her, give her a brilliant Christmas – just in case.

It was a good time. We went out to dinner, saw friends and took it easy. We spent as much time as we could at home, cuddling and watching TV and going for walks and snuggling up in bed. We made love for the first time since the operation. I began to feel like a young man again instead of a lone-ball, brain-damaged cancer survivor.

At work, there was plenty to do. I edited books pages, wrote film reviews and articles for the arts pages, complied the Friday 'What's On?' section of the paper, sorted out poetry submissions for the 'New Verse' slot and caught up on all the work I'd missed.

Most of the time I forgot all about hospitals and cancer.

In February I went back to Vincent's for three days of tests. On Friday morning I went straight from hospital to work. In the afternoon, Kate phoned me. Her soft voice was unusually light and carefree. For some reason, there was nobody in the office except me. 'I've some startling news,' she said.

I knew that something dreadful was coming because 'startling' was not a word that Kate ever used. She told me the cancer had come back. There were specks on my lungs and lymph nodes. It was likely that I would have to have treatment. But I wasn't to worry, she said. It meant that we'd have a couple of days in Liverpool out of it. There was a really fine sperm deposit clinic there and we could fly over tomorrow or the day after.

One side of my face became hot, as though it had been slapped. I didn't know what to say about anything. The numb feeling returned. Kate and I talked quietly for a few minutes. She was soothing and loving, almost crying. But I was too confused to reason things out, and I was mean and surly with her. I told her I'd phone her back.

I went to the window and opened it. My office was on the first floor. A van was spewing smoke as it pulled away from the pavement below where it had been making a delivery. The only coherent thought that came into my mind was that fucking fumes from those fucking vans had probably given me cancer. For a few moments, I despised all van drivers.

I got through the rest of the day by tearing into my work. I told my colleague, Colm, who had looked after my workload and arranged to have my mail delivered to me in hospital, that 'my little problem had returned'. Then I told my editor, Michael. Both were calm and reassuring. If they were shocked, they didn't let on. I was shocked enough for all of us.

At home, Kate and I sat up most of the night and tried to talk the whole thing out. I was still upset. She had to take a lot of shit.

Gradually, I improved. But I couldn't cry, even though I knew it would unclog a lot of fear and perhaps even assuage the savage anger rising in me that was seeking someone or something to blame. I felt that I had somehow brought it all on myself for the way I'd lived in the past – in my wild youth, my student drinking phase and my crazy rock-and-roll days.

Kate disappeared into the front room and put on one of our favourite records, Peter Gabriel's 'Don't Give Up', a moving duet between Gabriel and Kate Bush. The song's fragile opti-mism and message of love took me by surprise, and I cried.

It all gushed out. Kate held me while I sobbed into my hands. I didn't want Kate to see me bawling like a baby, so I kept my palms over my face until the wetness made them stick to my cheeks.

I cried for an hour. All my selfish fears were in the tears. I was going to die. I was going to be taken from Kate. I was never going to write the books I wanted or achieve any of the goals I had set myself. We were never going to have kids, raise a family, buy a house, take holidays, move to America or explore Paris again. We were never going to kiss, make love, have dreams, giggle, cuddle up in bed, go out, make dinners, have fights and make up, buy presents for each other, celebrate our love affair and all of its little anniversaries, hold hands on the beach in Cape Cod... why did it have to happen to me? To us? Someone was messing with the voodoo doll again.

I remained seated at the kitchen table, my elbows gouging into the wood. Kate stood beside me all the while, holding me into her and talking softly, telling me to cry and keep on crying, that there was nothing wrong with crying and we were going to be all right. She told me that it was unfair but that we had beaten the brain haemorrhage and we were going to beat this too.

When I couldn't cry anymore, we made coffee and talked. The cancer was spreading very fast, the oncologist had told Kate. Treatment had to begin within a few days. There was a chance that I would be infertile afterwards, so we had to decide quickly about Liverpool.

We argued for a while. In the end, I decided that I was going to need all my strength to kill off the cancer. Going to Liverpool to leave a sperm deposit would be like admitting that I might not make it through. As well as that, I didn't feel that you could make beautiful babies by going into a room in a clinic and jerking off into a tube. We'd have babies, I promised Kate. I knew it and I felt it.

As far as I was concerned, I was going to win. From then on, everything was going to be positive. I wanted to have treatment immediately – whatever it turned out to be. I wanted to start fighting.

Kate accepted that. We were going to beat this disease, together.

We rang Dr Maeve, who had been in touch with Kate earlier that morning. She was glad to hear that I was ready for immediate treatment. 'We're looking at chemotherapy,' she told me.

The prospect of chemotherapy scared me more than cancer. What did it do to you? I had heard that it meant months and months of agony. It made all your hair fall out, that was for sure.

While we were considering all of this, two friends arrived unexpectedly. They had been in the area and thought they would drop in. We met them downstairs and explained the situation. They apologised and went off.

But the visit of our friends calmed us. It brought back the everyday babble of life, where people called in on you, phoned up just to gossip, communicated about normal things. It made me feel like an ordinary person.

It helped us get through the night.

★

My mother knew something was wrong the moment I arrived unannounced at her door in Rathmines. She led me into the sitting room and sat down while I remained standing. Keeping my voice as steady and sharp as I could, I told Mother that I had something to say to her but that I didn't want her to start crying or shout or get hysterical or anything like that. She said that she wouldn't. Then I told her that I had cancer.

I told her that I was being treated in hospital but that I didn't want any visitors at all, except for Kate. Most important of all, I wanted her to promise me that she wouldn't tell Dad. I wanted to tell him myself, later. She promised, then sat and gazed at the floor for a while before asking me if I would like a cup of tea.

No thanks, I said. I have to go. I left as quickly as I could.

★

Professor Fennelly was the oncologist in charge of my case. A big, bustling man with an easy, friendly manner, he was also refreshingly straightforward.

He told me that testicular cancer was one of the most treatable forms of the disease. Apparently, the incidence of this particular cancer had doubled in Ireland over the past couple of years – no one knew why.

But it wasn't all bad news. If caught early enough, over ninety per cent of cases of testicular cancer could be totally cured. The main problem was that some guys didn't heed the swelling in their testes and carried on for six months or a year before seeking medical help. By that stage, it was often too late. The cancer would have spread, affecting the vital organs. Once that happened, treatment was both intensive and difficult, with no guarantee of success. A lot of guys had played Machoman with fatal consequences. Nearly a third of Irish men who contracted testicular cancer died.

Mine had been caught within the first four months and Fennelly was optimistic about my chances.

Fennelly's assistant was Dr Maeve, a bespectacled young woman with long blonde curls who always seemed to be under pressure. She also reckoned that I had a better than average chance of being completely cured. She told me not to fret about chemo. It wasn't half as rough as it was made out to be.

The regime, as my course of treatment was termed, would last twelve weeks. Each Thursday or Friday I would be treated in the Day Care Centre on the second floor of St Vincent's. But every third weekend I would have to check in to hospital for four or five days and be hooked up to a continuous drip. It was the most intensive course of its kind.

The talk with the doctors reassured me, but I was still scared, though I tried not to let it show. I decided to arm myself.

The day before my first full weekend session of chemotherapy, I bought myself a Sony Walkman. We had very little money at the time, but I figured that music was a life-enhancing investment. Whenever bad thoughts invaded, I could drive them away with Bruce Springsteen, Tom Petty, Creedence, The Bangles, John Lee Hooker, Sonny Boy Williamson, Fats Domino, Joe Jackson, Sade, Mink Deville, John Fogerty, even The Beach Boys – anything that made me feel good. I tried to track down a tape of Gnidrolog (I'd sold off all my vinyl albums shortly after I'd got married) but not even my pals in Freebird Records could find one for me.

I arrived at St Vincent's for my first session on 17 February. I carried a briefcase that was filled with tapes, books, jotter, biros, toiletries and batteries. My first ever pair of pyjamas were in there too, along with a nightshirt, slippers and a folding toothbrush – all of which Kate had bought for me during my first stay. It was like I had prepared for a short war. Everything I packed was going to help me win.

I told my friends I was going into hospital for chemotherapy. Most were shocked. Some wanted to know what kind of cancer I had. I was afraid to tell them the truth. Testicular cancer sounded so shameful, as though I were about to lose my private parts altogether through some fault of my own. I didn't want people to think that I was about to become a eunuch. I didn't care to think too much about it myself.

For a while, I told people I had abdominal cancer. It was a more serious form of cancer, but somehow it sounded less threatening to my manhood.

I was also reluctant to tell people about my operation. It was far too intimate, and the experience was still terrifyingly fresh in my mind. It seemed to me that I'd barely had a chance to recover from the shock of losing a testicle and now I had to face up to a battle against cancer. I had to deal with chemotherapy as well, so I lied about that too.

In a short time, I adjusted. When people asked, I told them the truth – mostly. To disguise my anxiety, I said I had gone from stereo to mono with one foul swoop of the surgeon's blade. 'It was the unkindest cut of all,' I said.

★

Everyone in the hospital referred to chemotherapy as chemo, like a nickname for an old pal. The nurses assured me that I would handle it easily.

'It'll be no bother to a fine big fella like you,' Nurse Val told me.

'You're a lot luckier than a lot of people,' Nurse Mary said.

For my first weekend session, I was put in a six-bed, semi-private room on the fourth floor. My bed was nearest the window, overlooking a smooth green golf course. Some of the beds had screens around them. Those that were open contained patients that were asleep most of the time. From time to time a patient was wheeled to or from the operating theatre. There was very little chat, just the squeaking of beds.

Dr Maeve hooked me up to drips that were connected to transparent bags of medication on tall mobile silver stands on either side of the bed. It took a while to get accustomed to the discomfort, to the awkwardness of having to manipulate a pair of steel hat stands dragging behind me whenever I wanted to go to the bathroom.

The next morning the drips were changed. While Dr Maeve was inserting the delicate butterfly needle into one of the veins on my right hand, a large man in the bed opposite began to mumble complaints through an explosion of black beard. He was lying fully clothed. One of the nurses asked the Irish Rasputin if he'd like a cup of tea. 'I'd rather have a nice, big, black, creamy pint,' Rasputin whined, and then he winked at me.

I didn't return his wink. As soon as I was hooked up, I slid the earphones over my head and pressed the play button.

Rasputin spent a day roaming the ward, moaning to any-one who'd listen. He affected a good humour, but I could feel his pessimism. He seemed to be trying to bring people down to his own level of despair.

That weekend, I instinctively avoided all those patients that had long faces on them. If a gloomy type approached I made sure to be deep in Walkman nirvana. It wasn't that I was cold or uncaring, it was simply a question of survival. I needed all my strength to fight my own battle.

As long as I remained optimistic, I could beat the cancer.

★

The word 'cancer' had a powerful effect on some patients. I heard stories about sufferers who were diagnosed and gave up the fight almost immediately. There was a story going around about a man who had died within three weeks of being told. Sometimes it was the word that killed people as much as the disease.

That was not going to happen to me. I would never give up and simply slide away.

I used everything I could – music, books, paintings and humour – to keep myself in a positive frame of mind. It was crucial to stay 'up' and be optimistic. The chemo would kill the cancer, but I felt that it needed help from the patient.

Whenever I sagged the nurses kept my spirits up. Nurse Mary, with whom I had made friends during my first stay, reminded me how important willpower was. 'I've seen people beat cancers that were a lot worse than yours. They just kept on fighting,' she told me.

In between offering advice and telling me stories, Nurse Mary liked to borrow books from me. She always read them in a night and returned them the next morning. Before the end of my first full session, I was loaning her books in batches of three or four.

At night I lay back in the sheets and imagined swarms of multicoloured, video-game Pacmen rushing along my blood-stream to gobble up all the cancer cells. I put all my repressed anger and hatred into the jaws of those little Pacmen.

But it was difficult to get a full night's sleep, even with the use of sleeping pills. Four or five times a night I had to get up, organise my trailing drip stands and pad over to the bathroom to relieve my super-sensitive bladder. To get into the bathroom, I had to nudge open the door with a combination of head and knee and then trundle everything past.

It was like being inside a spaceship, waiting for lift off. The bathroom glowed with orange light and there was a dull hum from underneath. Squatting or standing, I couldn't hear any of the snores or sobs or sighs or occasional long, dribbly farts from the ward.

By the fourth night I was sufficiently adept at manoeuvring my medical appendages to be able to leave cumbersome drip stands outside. By gently resting the edge of the door against the drip stand's narrow tube, the steady flow was maintained. I sat there holding my arm straight out in front of me so that the needle wouldn't pop out of my vein.

Most of the time I got back to bed without yanking the tube out or clogging it with blood.

★

At first I resisted making friends with the patients in the ward. It wasn't hard. There was a high turnover of patients and I rarely saw the same face twice.

In Day Care the following week, it was easy to remain immersed in a book or lost in Walkman music. I arrived at nine each morning and was hooked up to the drip before eleven. I was usually totally absorbed in my own universe by midday.

One day I was next to the bed of an old lady who sobbed and

muttered softly to herself. The screens were around her most of the time, even when visitors came. She had a lot of visitors. She gave them all the same detailed account of her ailments and symptoms and told them that it was the will of God that she was going. For some reason, her faltering voice cut through the music in my earphones. Between visitors, her sobs made everyone in the ward restless and uneasy.

After a time, most of her visitors made their excuses and shot from the room like arrows released from a strongbow. When my treatment finished and I was getting ready to leave, I could still hear her frail, trembling voice telling her tale of woes to one of the nurses. The nurse calmed the old lady down, humoured her and gave her hope.

During my second weekend session Nurse Val introduced me to a lively young woman who had been on chemo for a while. The woman was losing her long hair in tufts, but she wasn't worried. 'I'm going to buy a wig,' she joked. 'Which do you think? A red one or a green one? I've always wanted green hair.'

She said she was going to buy a special wig catalogue and pick the most hideous. She'd come and show me, she promised.

When Kate visited, Professor Fennelly and Dr Maeve told us that my blood count was near normal. The chemo was working. It was wiping out the cancer.

Kate was excited and relieved by the news. I was glad too, but it didn't mean as much to me. I remembered the way that I had felt in the office at work the day Kate had phoned to tell me the 'startling news'. I didn't want any more shocks. Once the treatment ended and I was cured, then I'd see about feeling euphoric.

★

I didn't really know what to expect from chemo. The first few sessions were easy. The only immediate effects were a slight weakness, numb toes and a lot of wind. Sometimes, walking along, I belched like an old toad. But I was warned that I would very soon be weak and nauseous, possibly depressed. Chemo affected everyone differently. The only sure thing was that my hair was going to fall out.

That was something I could handle.

One lunchtime shortly after my first full chemo session, I called to the Dublin Barber's on the quays next to the Virgin Megastore. I requested a crew cut, US Marine style. The Dublin Barber turned out to be an exuberant young Belfast man. He burbled with delight. 'Great. I've always wanted to do one of these.'

A couple of weeks later, I was taking a bath at home when I noticed a lot of black hairs floating in the water. The hair on my scalp felt brittle. It cracked in my fingers like tiny strands of dry spaghetti. Soon there was a swamp of black hair floating beside me.

At lunchtime the next day, I was back at the Dublin Barber's. 'Shave it off,' I told him. 'Every bit.'

'I've been waiting years for someone to say that,' the Dublin Barber said. The barber seemed to have the same response to everything. I got the impression that nothing phased him, not even giving a baldy haircut to a bloke who was going through chemo.

For the first few weeks of my baldness, I wore a black beret whenever I went outside. It made me look a little like a French painter, but it covered my bare skull and made me feel secure.

At work, I kept the beret on indoors at all times. I was too embarrassed to meet people without it on. At first, few of my colleagues knew what was wrong with me. Many were puzzled by my wearing a beret indoors. Others thought I'd flipped. Those who knew – like Colm and the editor, Michael – said nothing.

Some had their own theories. Once, descending the back stairs, I overheard a conversation between two men below. 'That Mac Anna fellow was always a pretentious bollocks,' one guy said. His pal agreed. But they were both wrong – after the operation, I was now technically a bollock. I passed by the two guys and said nothing. I had never seen either man before.

I found it hard to get used to being hairless all over. Even the beret couldn't disguise the absence of my eyebrows. Catching sight of myself sometimes in shopfront mirror windows on the street, I was shocked by the pale shadowless face under the headgear. With the beret off, I looked like an escaped psychopath – but I sure saved a lot on razors.

After a while I came to terms with being a bald head, but I could not get used to feeling tired all the time. Chemotherapy kills the fast-producing and mutating cancer cells, but it can also kill off your energy. The simplest physical task became a major trial for me. Walking from Tara Street Dart Station to Independent House in Abbey Street took nearly everything I had. Typing a film review left my fingers numb and my arms dangling. It required a huge effort to interview a person for the arts page. My mind was as agile as ever, but my body performed in creaking slow motion and quit easily.

The full extent of my new weakened state was brought home to me one day six weeks or so after treatment began. I was walking home from Dalkey in a strong wind, carrying a newspaper. At the corner of our road I dropped the paper and it started to flutter away in the breeze. I tried to run the couple of yards to stand on it to prevent the pages from blowing away – but I couldn't move. By the time I had walked over and bent down, most of the paper had flown away. Shattered, I watched the rest fly off and then I walked slowly home.

I learned to ration my time and energies carefully. If I grew overtired at work, I simply went home. When I was too exhausted to walk, I took a taxi. I worked in short productive bursts, followed by long recuperative breaks.

Travelling anywhere by Dart or bus was wonderful. All I had to do was sit and watch and think. Walking became an ordeal, but the accomplishment of getting someplace lifted me.

Work was a great therapy too. It made me feel that I was still in control of an important aspect of my life. Getting through a working day meant that I was beating the cancer, kicking the shit out if it.

At home, I took up to three naps a day. I went to bed at eight o'clock. It was the only way I could continue to function. All I had to do was to rest my head on a pillow and I was gone. I will never forget the crushing emptiness I felt upon being the first home to a dark, cold apartment and being too exhausted to do anything except conk out on the sofa.

At night, I had no dreams. Rising in the morning was a real-life monster movie.

On our days off Kate and I often drove to the Killiney Castle Hotel to go swimming in the heated indoor pool. In the water, I forgot my bald, hairless state. It was easy to swim and splash about like a youngster. It required a lot less effort than walking or typing up an article.

In the upstairs changing rooms, I towelled down in the corner with my back to the other men. I didn't want anyone to spot that I had only one testicle.

One day I noticed a small boy staring severely at me. The boy put his finger in his mouth and tugged at his father's togs. 'Da, look at your man, he's a skinhead.'

'Sssssh,' the father said and looked mortified.

The boy chewed his finger for a few moments. 'God, I'd hate to look like him,' he said.

I smiled at the father to show him that I wasn't going to throw his son out of the window – though I wanted to. The father made sure that his boy kept his beak shut after that probably in case I changed my mind.

Driving home, I told Kate about the incident and we

laughed. It doesn't do to take yourself too seriously all the time, no matter what's wrong with you. Kids are a great leveller.

Word got out about my illness. At work, certain people began avoiding me. Occasionally, I turned a corner to catch a glimpse of someone diving into a doorway, any doorway, or hastily turning on the stairs to zoom back the way they had come. I got the impression that some guys thought they could catch cancer from me or contract whatever fatal illness they'd heard that I was carrying merely by passing by me in a corridor.

Mostly, though, things were fine. People saw that I was fighting and they let me get on with it. For the most part, I was left alone at work. It was good to feel trusted. I wasn't given anything extra to do. I handled my normal workload, which was as much as I could cope with.

Some afternoons Ritchie and I met for coffee. We usually chose Sherries or somewhere quiet where we wouldn't run into people we knew. Ritchie told me what was going on in the world. I described the horrors of chemotherapy. I got the better deal.

Once, walking slowly back to work through the alleyway next to Wynn's Hotel, I pulled off my beret to joke that I had lost all of my hair, my eyebrows, my sense of smell and my left ball as well as nearly all my dignity. 'I must have done something terrible in a previous incarnation.'

'What do you mean "in a previous incarnation"?' Ritchie said.

★

As the weeks went on I began to look forward to the long stretches in hospital. In a way, the hospital stays relieved me of the responsibility for my illness. In a ward, I always felt surrounded and buoyed up by goodwill. It was as though every single doctor, nurse, orderly, ward sister and admin secretary was rooting for me to make it and be cured.

'You look crap. What's up with you?' Nurse Val asked me one day. I told her I felt weak and nauseous. 'Ah, you'll be all right. There's a lot worse off than you.'

Nurse Val was right. There were many people with more severe illnesses. I saw them in the hospital corridors every day, and sometimes in the bed next to mine. They made me feel blessed that my cancer had been caught in its early stages.

One of the best things about being in St Vincent's was that I could talk about cancer without feeling guilty or paranoid. In hospital, I didn't feel like a freak. Outside hospital, it was almost impossible to discuss my illness. At the mention of the word 'cancer', people grew uneasy and either changed the subject or found an excuse to leave. It got to the point where I began to feel ashamed for having cancer. My cancer was dirty, uncivilised, bad manners, impolite, disgusting, contagious, fatal and unpleasant. It reminded some people of their own frail mortality. It made me avoid people whenever possible.

Eventually and through no effort of mine, I became friends with Shay, another cancer patient. Shay wasn't put off by my coolness or by my attempts to seclude myself in books or my Walkman. 'Lost a bit on top, I see,' he said the first time we met.

I laughed and replied that I had, but that his own thatch didn't look too safe.

Shay had lymphoma. This was his second bout of chemo. His fair hair now stood out in wispy tufts. He didn't want to shave it. His kids would pull it out for him, he said. That would save him the cost of a barber.

Shay was a gentle and optimistic guy. It was good to talk to someone in the same predicament that was good humoured and hopeful. He made me feel foolish for having isolated myself so much. At Day Care treatment I usually took the bed across from him. We discussed news and world events and we

swapped tapes. He gave me jazz and classical. I gave him country rock and blues.

On the long weekends I chatted to the nurses and began to
open up with the other patients. Whenever I got tired, though,
I went back to hiding in music or books.

Sometimes I was placed in a window bed. I watched the golfers
on the course outside. They teed off from a spot directly below.
They had a clear view across acres of long, rolling, uninterrupt-
ed green. They couldn't miss. The only obstacle was a small
clump of trees to their extreme right. I lost count of the number
of golfers who shot into the trees. I lay on my bed, giggling as I
watched these frumpy incompetents in loud jackets and striped
shoes whacking around in the branches with their clubs, searching for their lost golf balls – which usually stayed lost.

On my third long weekend in St Vincent's, Joe was admitted
and given the bed next to mine. Joe was in for tests. There was
something wrong with his lungs, but nobody knew what exactly. A special oxygen mask was attached to the wall beside him.
Every couple of hours he placed it over his nose and mouth
and breathed in and out. He made rattling, clanking wheezes,
like a knight in armour climbing stairs.

Joe was a quiet Dub with a thick, black moustache and a freck-
led, earnest face. He worried a lot about his family, his health
and work. I lent him books and I told him funny stories about
what it was like to have a suddenly bald head. His family came
to see him every day. The kids were as quiet and gentle as their
father. I never saw them run about or heard them shout and I
never heard them raise their voices. Joe's elegant, dark-haired
wife sat by his side. Joe and his wife spoke in soft, unhurried
voices. The kids too, sat by their father's bedside for as long as
visiting hours would allow. The family couldn't have Joe at
home, so they brought their home in to him. When visiting time
was up, they left quietly and without fuss. Joe always got up and
walked them to the lifts.

He was fascinated by the needles and tubes going into my arms and hand, as well as by the drip stands. He couldn't get over the fact that I had to drag those monsters behind me whenever I left my bed.

One morning he told me that he had experienced dreadful nightmares since arriving in hospital, until one night when he awoke to see my domed figure emerging from the bathroom in my striped nightshirt, with gleaming steel drip stands behind. In the orange glow of the open bathroom doorway, I was Frankenstein's monster rising from the cellar.

After that, Joe's nightmares went away. They just couldn't compete with reality.

★

At work, I avoided the canteen. I ventured upstairs to the main news and features subbing areas only when it was absolutely necessary or if I had copy to deliver. I continued to wear the beret indoors, as though it were a magical shield.

The writer Dermot Bolger called in to my office one afternoon to drop off a book review. I called him The Moving Beard. He called me Freckles McVinnie (people were always taking liberties with my name). He commented on my beret, so I told him about my cancer. 'Whip it off and give us a look at your bald head,' he said.

I took off my beret. Dermot produced a small camera. 'Got to get a shot of this.'

He grabbed someone from the corridor and asked them to take a picture of the two of us. The Moving Beard and Bald Head posed alongside a typewriter. Both of us smiled at the camera.

After that, I decided that it was stupid and cowardly to wear a disguise. I got into the habit of taking the beret off once I was seated at my desk. I was bald and odd looking, but so what?

Lots of others were weirder looking than me and they weren't sick. At least I had an excuse.

However, the chemo had made me weak. I was also super-sensitive. The casual slights of life got to me in a way that they never had before.

One afternoon I was talking to a friend in the street outside my office building when a Designer Anorak with a receding hairline who knew of my condition came around the corner. 'Ah, come out of the closet, have we?' he said good naturedly, slapping me heartily on the back as he bustled past.

I was shocked, but I was also hurt and angry. What fucking closet? Did he mean that I should stay home and not show my bald head or hairless state until I was cured – or dead? 'At least my hair's going to grow back,' I yelled as the Anorak scooted around another corner.

I don't think that he heard me. Yelling after him made me feel better. As soon as I calmed down, I realised that Anorak Man hadn't meant any harm. He was just one of life's jolly-natured insensitives.

★

At movie press screenings I took my usual place in the front rows. I kept my beret on while the film was rolling. I was worried that my bald head would gleam in the projection flicker. It was late April before I got the confidence to sit through a movie with my cap off.

Most nights I came home from work too knackered to do anything except nap and watch TV.

Cancer cropped up everywhere.

Former champion jockey Jonjo O'Neill was interviewed about his cancer on a BBC awards programme. He was now a bald head and he was still on chemo. His calm resolution cheered me.

Dr Vicky Clement-Jones appeared on *Wogan*. Five years previously she had been diagnosed with terminal cancer and given two months to live. She was still going strong. Her gentle philosophical spirit gave me great hope.

To amuse Kate I sang along with the TV ad jingles. The Bisto Kids was my favourite. It was childish carry-on, but it brought me joy.

Anything that brought joy was fine with me.

★

The only major outing I made during chemo was to Paul Simon's Graceland gig at the RDS.

Ritchie arranged the tickets and my colleague Frank picked me up at home and drove me there. Inside the enormous dark hall, Frank remained close by me in case I fell over suddenly or exploded or lost an arm or leg.

It was uplifting to be in the midst of an excited crowd. Such a big deal to be out in the world, doing something as normal as going to a concert.

At one stage I went off to buy Cokes. A rock concert is one of the few places on earth where an odd appearance doesn't look out of place. Nobody stared at the spaces above my eyes where my eyebrows should have been or commented on my beret as I queued up at the drinks stand. Getting back to Frank and Ritchie and Colm with the Cokes was a big achievement. Just a simple everyday thing, but it meant a lot to me.

Paul Simon sang with delicate sincerity. I could feel the music filling me with strength. Every couple of numbers or so, Simon gave up the stage to the South African artists and musicians that he had collaborated with in the making of his *Graceland* album. Some among the audience were disappointed. They wanted Simon to sing his hits all night.

I couldn't understand that. I had never seen an act as

appealing as Ladysmith Black Mambaza, a ten-piece acapella group that sang with captivating precision and style. They moved and harmonised with such simple joy they made me want to dance – that would probably have finished me off.

Towards the end of the evening Hugh Masekela came on. He sang with gravelly authority. He played glorious, shrilling trumpet on 'Coal Train', the story of the tragic plight of the migrant black workers who worked in the mines in South Africa. It was powerful as well as passionate. It was not the music of despair or defeat and it exhilarated me.

I had a wonderful time. It was the only time during my illness when I almost forgot that I had cancer.

Just before the encores I suddenly became very tired and had to leave. I told Frank that I would catch a taxi outside, but he insisted on driving me to my door. 'Yarrah, sure, I was going that way anyhow,' he said in his soft Cork burr.

★

My life became extremely simple.

Everything was reduced to basics. I let my instincts influence my dealings with people. Pessimists were bad; optimists were good. If someone annoyed or disturbed me I stayed away from them. If someone was kind I lapped it up and added it to my reserves of strength.

At some stage I got a phone call from John Sutton to ask if I would read a manuscript of a novel about a rock band by Roddy Doyle, who I remembered from college days. As I'd been a rock and roller, John thought I might be the very man to check the accuracy of the rock-music details. I said OK, and the next day the manuscript arrived on my desk.

It was a fortnight before I got around to reading *The Commitments*. I really enjoyed the book and I phoned John to say that I would be happy to meet with Roddy. But I was sick a lot and Roddy was busy so it was a week or longer before we could agree a time and place to meet.

We met in Bewley's and I handed him back his manuscript. I told him the rock stuff was sound and that I had really enjoyed the book. I may have added that the novel was a bit short. I saw him looking at my beret and my hairless eyebrows. I'm sure he guessed what was up with me, but he was too polite to say anything. We wished each other well.

Afterwards, walking back to the newspaper, I felt jaded and suddenly frustrated. I wanted to be writing books too. I had attempted several novels and short stories, but they had been poor. I had even tried to write a novel about a rock band, but had given up after three chapters. Now that I was in cancer limbo, I couldn't do anything. I wanted this cancer shite to be over. I wanted my life back.

Occasionally I caught someone looking at me with stone-dead eyes, as though dismissing my chances. I had Kate to comfort me, and there was still good news from Professor Fennelly concerning my blood tests and x-rays. The cancer had been gone since mid-March. It should be well and truly killed off by the time my chemo regime finished in May.

Home days and nights were quiet. The phone rarely rang. People left us alone. Some were scared, many were unsure about what to say to a person who had cancer. There were a few – like the ones who gave me the stone-eyed looks – that believed that anyone with cancer was a goner. I might beat it this time, but it would be back for certain. To some people, I was a dead man – that was hard to get used to.

I went for walks as often as I could. Short walks. To Bullock Harbour and Dalkey town, both ten minutes from where we lived. I loved to stand on the pier at Bullock and toss coins into the sea. I wished for good things. I asked God to help me beat the cancer for ever.

In Dalkey I liked to browse through the shelves of second-hand books in the Exchange bookshop. I often bought a *Herald* and went to Georgina's Delicatessen for a coffee and danish.

Simple adventures. But they made me feel good.

★

My final session of chemo was rough. I suffered from dreadful nausea and vomited so often and fiercely into the silver dish beside my bed that I thought I had spewed up part of my stomach. My veins had all but collapsed. It took a great deal of patient and meticulous struggle before a nurse could insert the drip needles into my arm.

During my last afternoon in Day Care a young doctor had just managed to complete the difficult process of hooking me up when there was a sudden *thunk* at the window that made us both jump. A golfer had accidentally teed off in the direction of the hospital. The young doctor was unperturbed. 'Happens now and again, I wouldn't worry about it,' he said.

Later one of the nurses told me that the year before a golf ball had come through a third-floor window. I had a sudden vision of beating cancer only to be assassinated by a wayward drive from a lunatic golfer. I would end up as a bizarre headline in my own newspaper.

Nurse Val came to say goodbye. She was off to Perth in Australia. She might stay there, she didn't know yet. Anyway, she promised to send me a postcard. I told her I'd write to her. 'You'll be grand,' she said. 'You're doing really well.'

At the beginning of May I was pronounced 'cured'. Professor Fennelly told me that I was now in full remission. I was now what was termed 'ninety-six per cent cured'. It meant that I had a ninety-six per cent chance of never having cancer again.

I wrote it in my diary at work. 'Ninety-six per cent cured.'

Fennelly told me that by Christmas I could even have a full head of hair.

Like an eejit, I thought it was really over.

Back at work, I told people I was cured and plunged into my job. I wanted to make up for lost time. I even left the beret at home.

However, my strength failed to return. Instead of getting back to full health, I grew paler and more nauseous by the day.

Within a week I was having trouble walking. My weight went down and I had constant headaches. I couldn't understand it. What was happening to me? Was this what it was like to feel 'ninety-six per cent cured'?

I certainly didn't feel particularly cured.

One morning I was assigned to write a colour feature about the adventures of a busload of American visitors as they toured Dublin. I had difficulty focusing on the page while taking notes. By lunchtime I was flagging. I had no energy, I couldn't catch my breath. A young American tourist came up to me with concern on her face. 'I don't mean to disturb you,' she said, 'but do they have chicken wings in Ireland?'

On Wednesday, 18 May, less than two weeks after my final chemo, I finished my film reviews and tried to write the colour feature. I couldn't do it. The words would not come and I couldn't think clearly. I left work early. I felt feverish and drained.

The next morning, I couldn't hold down food. I had violent eruptions of pain in my sides and back. It was like being stuck with hot needles. My bowels felt like I had bricks inside me. I couldn't drink a glass of water without puking. I couldn't eat, couldn't crap and couldn't even walk.

For the first time since I had fallen ill, I actually considered the possibility that I wasn't going to make it.

Kate sent for the doctor again. This time he sent me to hospital immediately. While I was packing my pyjamas, the doctor told Kate that he thought the cancer could have spread to my liver, which would mean it was terminal. Kate didn't panic or cry. She organised me and led me to the car. Bald head knew that he was banjaxed again, but he didn't know why. He was too sick to even think about it.

'Please don't turn on the radio,' Bald head said. 'I don't want to hear fucking *West Side* Fucking *Story*.'

At the hospital, the nurses couldn't believe that I was back. Some didn't recognise the pale, skinny, hairless, lurching ancient in the dressing gown and slippers who had to be helped from the car to the lift.

I was put in bed and a nurse drew the screens. I didn't object. The fever was making me dizzy and I had almost no strength left to talk.

I had no funny cracks to amuse the nurses, none for myself. I just wanted to stop being sick. My back and chest had broken out in sore red spots that wouldn't let me get comfortable in the bed. Whenever I made a move, my sides exploded in sudden pain.

Dr Bloodhound came to visit me and was polite to me. That's it, I thought. I'm finished now.

A nurse gave me some pills to ease the fever. Then Professor Fennelly came around to examine me. He checked the area round my liver and told me I would be fine. He seemed relieved.

Then he took Kate outside into the corridor for a private chat.

When Kate returned she had that tight look on her face again. 'You'll be fine love,' she said. 'You're just completely run down.'

I didn't believe a word.

I thought I was a dead man.

★

I didn't have liver cancer.

But I did have pneumonia, pleurisy, chronic anaemia and a stack of minor ailments.

The chemo had seriously weakened my immune system and I had been attacked by everything that was going. I had tried to resume a normal working life too soon after my 'cure'. Now I was paying the price.

My body was very seriously run down and I needed complete rest.

The brain haemorrhage hadn't killed me.

Neither had the cancer.

Nor even the chemo.

But the side effects were having a fair shot at it.

It didn't seem that I would ever be well again. I was a practical joke. Whenever the gods of health had a medical experiment to conduct they chose me to be the guinea pig. It was humiliating.

I didn't even make jokes about voodoo dolls anymore. I just wanted it to be all over.

The next morning I was given intravenous antibiotics. That went on for a couple of days and nights. Then, just as I was feeling at my weakest, Mother came to visit me.

I had been dozing when I heard my name being called. I opened my eyes to find that Mother was standing in front of me. She was dressed from head to toe in black and had her back to me. She was staring at the guy in the bed opposite who was also bald and tall and dishevelled looking. 'Ferdia, is that you?'

Mother advanced towards the guy in the other bed with her arms out. She was distraught and she began to sob as she said my name again.

The guy in the other bed had been reading a magazine. He looked up to find a strange, sobbing woman dressed like the angel of death heading towards him with her arms out. He must have thought that his time on earth was up. His eyes opened wide and he went pale and dropped the magazine.

'Mother, I'm over here,' I called.

Mother stopped and slowly turned around. The guy in the

other bed looked relieved. 'Oh Ferdia,' she said and came towards me with her arms out.

Mother was really distraught. She had found out that I had gone back into hospital and immediately presumed the worst. She was going to stay with me till I got better. It was her duty, she said.

I could see that this visit wasn't going to do either of us any good. I calmed her down as best I could. I told her I was getting better, but that she would have to go. I wasn't well enough for visitors yet. I'd call her soon, I promised.

Somehow, I managed to get to my feet. Trailing drip stands, I escorted Mother to the lifts. I made sure she got inside and then I waved goodbye to her as the doors closed. As the lift descended I heard her sobbing loudly, and also complaining that her own son had thrown her out of the hospital. The sobbing faded away as the lift descended.

I was about to drag the drip stands and myself back to my room, but something made me stay.

A few moments later, Mother's voice faded up again, as though someone was turning up a volume control. Her voice grew louder as the lift ascended. There was a soft bing as the lift stopped at my floor. The lift doors opened, revealing my mother in the midst of a bunch of other patients and visitors, all of whom were listening with the greatest sympathy to her story about being thrown out of hospital by her own sick son.

I gave Mother a hug and put her back into the lift, and pressed the button for the ground floor. This time she went home.

★

After a couple of days, I felt a lot better. My colour returned. The bricks in my bowels dissolved. I started eating again. I didn't puke or feel nauseous. By the afternoon of the third day, I felt reborn.

I could feel summer coming.

'Good times on the way,' I told Kate. I sang her the silly Bisto Kids jingle.

I spent two slow and easy weeks in hospital. Then I took a month off work.

There was no stress anymore. No pressure. I dawdled about at home. I went off for long walks. I visited Georgina's and drank coffee. I read books, watched a lot of TV.

Jonjo showed up on a BBC sports programme and looked well. Dr Vicky Clement-Jones appeared on a late-night discussion on Channel Four, but she seemed tired and uninterested. I got a postcard from Nurse Val in Perth. She was doing brilliantly. She asked how I was, but she forgot to include her address.

I met Shay for a pint. He appeared well and healthy and his hair was growing back.

Kate and I made plans to take a long summer break on Cape Cod. We deserved a holiday. We needed one.

Dad came to Dalkey to see me. He was softly curt and stone faced. He sat on one of the wobbly kitchen chairs, a great dark sprawl of presence with cigarette ash trickling from his shoulder. He studied me with a softer, more inquisitive gaze now, as though he were discovering several new characteristics about the face and eyes of his troublesome oldest son. He gave me money to help towards the cost of the holiday and I thanked him. 'Don't thank me,' he said. 'Just buy your mother and me a castle sometime.'

Then he borrowed as many books as he could carry to his car with him and drove off.

★

On 3 August Kate and I boarded an Aer Lingus jumbo bound for Boston.

I had grown a spiky crew cut, slightly longer than US Marine style, and for the first time in nearly a year I felt healthy. Kate ordered champagne from the stewardess. I drank Ballygowan.

While the jet's engines warmed up for the takeoff, I read through the English newspapers. On page two of one of the broadsheets, a small one-paragraph news item announced the death from cancer of Dr Vicky Clement-Jones.

As I was showing the news item to Kate, the plane took off.

It's never really over.

Once a cancer survivor, always a cancer survivor.

Some patients make the adjustment back into normal life without too much trouble. At first I was confident that I would too.

But I didn't expect to have depressions that dogged me for months. The depressions often arose from petty frustrations or repressed anger at a perceived slight or nasty remark. Nor did I anticipate feeling so vulnerable in my dealings with people, especially those I thought had little sympathy or understanding for what I had gone through.

It took me a long time to shake off the cancer hangover, and in a way I never truly succeeded in letting go of it.

Fighting off depressions was something I could handle. I told myself that I got through a brain haemorrhage, cancer and a tough chemo regime, so the depression was minor by comparison.

And I was always aware that there were others far worse off.

There was still a fear that the cancer could return. The monthly blood tests I took for over a year after my treatment finished were a constant reminder.

But the fears lessened as the time passed. Once a year had gone without a recurrence, doctors assured us that it was virtually certain that I would be clear for the rest of my life.

Ninety-six per cent certain.

Around Christmas I got a phone call from one of Shay's friends. Shay had died that morning. The friend wanted to let me know because he knew that Shay and I had been close. I thanked the friend and put the phone down, and then I cried more deeply and for longer than I had ever cried in my life. I had presumed that Shay was going to make it. I had assumed that because we had both finished our chemo around the same time that we were both through and were now finished with cancer. I had been looking forward to meeting up with him for pints and chats and to swap music tapes.

I went to Shay's funeral, but I don't recall much about it. I don't think I stayed long. For a long time afterwards, I felt guilty that I had survived. A year after cancer, I was healthier than I had ever been. No matter how depressed I sometimes got, I never felt that the cancer was going to return.

★

I notice bald heads in the street all the time. Some choose to go bare headed. Other wear hats or even wigs. One or two sport berets.

But the lack of eyebrows is a real giveaway.

Once I saw a young bald head standing in the queue for the Pass machine outside the Bank of Ireland on the bridge end of O'Connell Street. He was bare headed. There were tiny blonde fluffs of hair dotted about his scalp. He wore a long green mac and he had an anxious expression on his keen, young features. He seemed to be daring people to look at him.

I passed and said nothing, though I felt a strong bond with him. I wished him good luck and a strong will. I hoped that he was as lucky as me and had someone who loved him enough to get him through it all. I hope that he had someone who would be waiting for him when it was all over.

Afterword

After cancer, my life got a lot simpler.

I rarely drank and for a long time I stayed home in the evenings. I became a bit of a recluse and that was when I started to write.

I looked forward to leading a normal life. At first my hair grew back curly and fair, but within a year it had started to recede. It remained long and straggly at the back, but disappeared up front. I was becoming a natural bald head. I was outraged. This was not in the script. My hair was supposed to return for good, not flit across my scalp on brief visits with more of it waving goodbye every couple of weeks.

I went to a barber to see if he could do something stylish with the bit that remained. 'How about a ponytail?' I suggested.

'How about a transplant?' he replied.

My hair continued to disappear. The only way to make it appear that I had any hair at all was to crop what there was into a merciless crew cut.

For a brief period in 1988 I was convinced that my sense of smell was returning, but I was just kidding myself. The brain haemorrhage had completely destroyed that part of my brain. The aromas that I thought I detected were merely ghosts in my nostrils, memories triggered by the sight of food cooking on a pan or a walk along the seashore. I can distinguish strong odours – I always know when I'm passing a rubbish tip – but I can't tell what is making them or where they are coming from. I miss the scent of perfume and I even miss not being able to smell garlic.

I saw a lot more of my parents. Dad developed a habit of calling in on me unexpectedly, ostensibly to borrow books but really to see how I was doing. He rarely sat down and usually left within twenty minutes, having borrowed about half a dozen of my books. He feigned disinterest in my condition, but I occasionally caught him giving me one of his deep, studious looks where he checked to see if any further bits of his eldest had fallen off or looked suspicious. I envied the fact that he had more hair than me.

I gave him books for Christmas and Dad often gave me a book as a birthday present. A year after my recovery from cancer, Dad gave me a book for my birthday that looked oddly familiar. On the book's inside page Dad had written, 'To Ferdia, Happy Birthday, X Dad.' However, on the next page I found a familiar scrawl: 'To Dad, Happy Christmas, X Ferdia'.

Dad was still Mr Abbey Theatre and Mother was still his *speirbhean*. I have almost forgiven them for the Rock Hudson business.

★

Kate and I had one more shock to face.

Soon after I recovered from cancer, a doctor told us that there was a good chance that we would never have kids. I was still trying to feel my way back into everyday life after cancer and a brain haemorrhage and now here was this new crisis. I had never really thought about children before. I had rushed headlong through my life, rarely pausing long enough for reflection, particularly during my rock-and-roll years or afterwards. Now I had a job, a good marriage and my health back. I also had all the time I would ever need to consider the prospect of a life without kids, a prospect that made me feel empty and unfulfilled. I developed a yearning for children and family life, something I had never once thought about before.

I didn't like being told that I might not have kids. As far as I was concerned, it was only a 'might', not a definite prognosis. Still, it caused deep concern and distress. I felt sad for Kate. Her Irish husband had survived falling to ribbons for three years and now it looked like he might be infertile. The crises that began almost immediately after our wedding were set to continue indefinitely. The world doesn't cut you a break just because you have been through a tough time.

Even the holidays in Cape Cod couldn't completely lift the sense of loss. On a sandy beach on a gloriously sunny day with nothing to do but eat ice cream and swim and sunbathe, it was hard to totally lose a recurring pang of hopelessness.

Then something strange but wonderful occurred. I cannot explain what happened – and I have no particular belief in the supernatural or the magical – but the events made me believe that everything would work out all right. In fact, there were two occurrences.

The first happened on the beach at Chatham in Cape Cod during the summer of 1989. I was watching Kate walk back along the water's edge when suddenly I saw the face of a young blonde girl in her face. It seemed to me that my wife was being accompanied by a little blonde girl. I don't know how else to describe it, nor can I explain why I felt certain that a child was coming to us, but I knew it with the same assurance that you have when you feel raindrops on your skin and accept that it's about to rain. We were going to have a little blonde girl.

I told Kate about my strange 'vision' and she was delighted. She seemed to accept that it would happen. The following year, Kate became pregnant and I felt a glowing inner confidence. But we suffered a miscarriage and I doubted my 'vision' for a long time. I thought that I must have been deluded.

Then, a year and a half year later, our daughter Sisi (Sienna) was born. I was present at the birth and the nurse handed me a pair of scissors to let me cut the umbilical cord and even though I only made one (I thought) simple snip, I still managed to leave blood splatters all over the ceiling. The room looked like a scene from *Nightmare on Elm Street*. 'The ward sister is not going to like that in the morning,' the nurse said.

In recent years, I have often watched Sisi walking along the beach in Cape Cod with Kate, just as I had seen in the 'vision' years ago. Sisi is blonde and tall and elegant. I always feel a terrific surge of uplift and joy. The first time I saw the real image of mother and daughter on the beach, I felt that I had been given the greatest benefits that life has to offer – children of our own and family life.

Two years after Sisi was born, I had another unexplainable 'vision'. I was looking out of our bathroom window late one night. In the strong moonlight I could clearly see our swings at the bottom of the garden where a little blonde girl was playing with a smaller, dark-haired boy.

In the morning I told Kate we were going to have another child and it would be a dark-haired boy. We were thrilled when she became pregnant again. On St Patrick's Day Kate gave birth to a little blonde girl, Bessa. We now had two little girls in our family, and it felt wonderful.

A year and a half later late got pregnant again. We had another baby, a boy with dark hair. I realised that I had already seen Sisi in the first 'vision' that day on the beach on Cape Cod. In the second 'vision' I had seen our daughter, Bessa, playing in the garden with her younger brother, Finn. I watched that scene in the garden for real many times over the years.

These were the only out-of-the-ordinary 'visions' that I have ever experienced.

Now we live in a good house in Sandycove, just across the bay from the old bungalow in Howth where my family lived for nearly three decades from the sixties. On a clear day I can still make out the roads in Howth where Nessan and I and various other friends rambled at weekends and during the summers that never seemed to end. I still feel a weird emotional attachment to the place that I can't explain. In my head Howth is still my home. I feel that I could live in Sandycove for a hundred years, but a part of me will always be a Howth 'runner-in'. I will always see home as the white-walled bungalow on Thormanby Road.

Occasionally, I go to my old hometown for a visit and I usually drive past my old home. The house is now an impressive two stories with tasteful pillars outside the front door. The garden looks different as well, though it's hard to tell from a moving car. The house is almost unrecognisable, but the driveway is still the same and the grassy bank where Naoise used to sit playfully tossing rocks into the traffic is almost unchanged. Tucked into the opposite bank and overhung with foliage at the bottom of the driveway there's a gate stump, a sole reminder of the white-painted wooden gates that Dad drove through one afternoon when I was fourteen. Somehow, with all the refurbishment and changes, a white-painted gate stump has survived.

The people who live in my old house have very graciously invited me to return to visit the place, but so far I haven't managed to pluck up the courage to accept the offer. Maybe one day I will.

Acknowledgements

I wish to thank Sheila O'Callaghan of RTÉ Radio for devising and producing *Teenage Kicks*, a series of radio documentaries that I wrote and presented on RTÉ Radio 1 in 2003.

My warmest regards to everyone at Hodder Headline Ireland. I am eternally grateful to Breda Purdue and Ciara Considine for commissioning and believing in this book and my huge thanks and appreciation to Claire Rourke for editing and encouraging.

I would also like to thank my parents, Tomás and Caroline, my sisters and brothers.

I am lucky to have had the love and support of my wife, Kate, and my children Sisi, Bessa and Finn.

My thanks and appreciation to my friend Seamus McClelland without whose keen sense of humour and perspective, not to mention an excellent memory, Johnny Jurex might never have happened.

I am grateful to Pat Butler for all his help with the Gaelige. I also wish to express my deepest thanks to Dermot Bolger who first gave me a voice.

Ferdia Mac Anna
September 2004

Permission Acknowledgements

The lines from 'Fern Hill' by Dylan Thomas, from *Collected Poems* published by Dent, are reproduced by kind permission of David Higham Associates.

Every effort has been made to fulfil requirements with regard to reproducing copyright material. the author and publisher will be glad to rectify any omissions at the earliest opportunity.